E. Carlos Rodríguez-Merchán
Editor

Advances in Revision Total Knee Arthroplasty

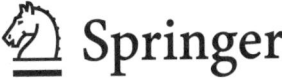

Editor
E. Carlos Rodríguez-Merchán
Department of Orthopedic Surgery
La Paz University Hospital
Madrid, Madrid, Spain

ISBN 978-3-031-60447-8   ISBN 978-3-031-60445-4 (eBook)
https://doi.org/10.1007/978-3-031-60445-4

© The Editor(s) (if applicable) and The Author(s), under exclusive license to Springer Nature Switzerland AG 2024

This work is subject to copyright. All rights are solely and exclusively licensed by the Publisher, whether the whole or part of the material is concerned, specifically the rights of translation, reprinting, reuse of illustrations, recitation, broadcasting, reproduction on microfilms or in any other physical way, and transmission or information storage and retrieval, electronic adaptation, computer software, or by similar or dissimilar methodology now known or hereafter developed.

The use of general descriptive names, registered names, trademarks, service marks, etc. in this publication does not imply, even in the absence of a specific statement, that such names are exempt from the relevant protective laws and regulations and therefore free for general use.

The publisher, the authors and the editors are safe to assume that the advice and information in this book are believed to be true and accurate at the date of publication. Neither the publisher nor the authors or the editors give a warranty, expressed or implied, with respect to the material contained herein or for any errors or omissions that may have been made. The publisher remains neutral with regard to jurisdictional claims in published maps and institutional affiliations.

This Springer imprint is published by the registered company Springer Nature Switzerland AG
The registered company address is: Gewerbestrasse 11, 6330 Cham, Switzerland

If disposing of this product, please recycle the paper.

Preface

Revision total knee arthroplasty (rTKA) is a surgical procedure that is being performed more and more frequently due to the longevity of the world's population. It is necessary when primary total knee arthroplasty (pTKA) fails for septic or aseptic reasons. It is a complex procedure in which there are still controversial issues.

In this book, expert authors on rTKA analyze the following chapters, which, as editor of this work, I have considered to be of the greatest interest: the burden of rTKA; the impact of tobacco use on rTKA outcomes; the impact of obesity on rTKA outcomes; the impact of preoperative opioid use on patient-reported outcomes after rTKA; assessment of patient satisfaction following rTKA; isolated versus full component revision in total knee arthroplasty for aseptic loosening; wound complications following rTKA; one-stage revision for periprosthetic joint infection (PJI); two-stage revision for PJI; rTKA for arthrofibrosis; rTKA for implant-related metal allergy; robotic-assisted rTKA; metal augments, polyethylene thickness, and stem length affect tibial baseplate load transfer in rTKA; cementless porous-coated metaphyseal sleeves used for bone defects in rTKA; chronic extensor mechanism failure after pTKA or rTKA: reconstructive and augmentation options; artificial intelligence in rTKA; and re-rTKA.

It is my wish and that of all the chapter authors that the contents of this book may help orthopedic surgeons engaged in performing such a difficult and complex surgical procedure as rTKA.

Madrid, Spain   E. Carlos Rodríguez-Merchán

Contents

1 **The Burden of Revision Total Knee Arthroplasty** 1
   E. Carlos Rodríguez-Merchán, Hortensia De la Corte-Rodríguez,
   and Juan M. Román-Belmonte

2 **The Impact of Tobacco Use on Revision Total Knee
   Arthroplasty Outcomes** 11
   E. Carlos Rodríguez-Merchán, Hortensia De la Corte-Rodríguez,
   and Juan M. Román-Belmonte

3 **The Impact of Obesity on Revision Total Knee Arthroplasty
   Outcomes** 17
   E. Carlos Rodríguez-Merchán, Hortensia De la Corte-Rodríguez,
   and Juan M. Román-Belmonte

4 **Impact of Preoperative Opioid Use on Revision Total Knee
   Arthroplasty Outcomes** 25
   E. Carlos Rodríguez-Merchán

5 **Patient Satisfaction After Revision Total Knee Arthroplasty** 37
   E. Carlos Rodríguez-Merchán

6 **Isolated Versus Full-Component Revision in Total Knee
   Arthroplasty for Aseptic Loosening** 43
   E. Carlos Rodríguez-Merchán

7 **Wound Complications Following Revision Total Knee
   Arthroplasty** 51
   E. Carlos Rodríguez-Merchán, Carlos A. Encinas-Ullán,
   Juan S. Ruiz-Pérez, and Primitivo Gómez-Cardero

8 **One-Stage Revision Total Knee Arthroplasty for Periprosthetic
   Joint Infection** 61
   E. Carlos Rodríguez-Merchán, Carlos A. Encinas-Ullán,
   Juan S. Ruiz-Pérez, and Primitivo Gómez-Cardero

9	Two-Stage Revision Total Knee Arthroplasty for Periprosthetic Joint Infection 73
	E. Carlos Rodríguez-Merchán, Carlos A. Encinas-Ullán, Juan S. Ruiz-Pérez, and Primitivo Gómez-Cardero
10	Revision Total Knee Arthroplasty for Arthrofibrosis 87
	E. Carlos Rodríguez-Merchán
11	Revision Total Knee Arthroplasty for Implant-Related Metal Allergy 95
	E. Carlos Rodríguez-Merchán
12	Robotic-Assisted Revision Total Knee Arthroplasty 105
	E. Carlos Rodríguez-Merchán, Carlos A. Encinas-Ullán, Juan S. Ruiz-Pérez, and Primitivo Gómez-Cardero
13	Metal Augments, Polyethylene Thickness, and Stem Length Affect Tibial Baseplate Load Transfer in Revision Total Knee Arthroplasty 111
	E. Carlos Rodríguez-Merchán
14	Cementless Porous-Coated Metaphyseal Sleeves Used for Bone Defects in Revision Total Knee Arthroplasty 121
	E. Carlos Rodríguez-Merchán, Carlos A. Encinas-Ullán, Juan S. Ruiz-Pérez, and Primitivo Gómez-Cardero
15	Chronic Extensor Mechanism Failure After Primary or Revision Total Knee Arthroplasty: Reconstructive and Augmentation Options. 129
	E. Carlos Rodríguez-Merchán, Carlos A. Encinas-Ullán, Juan S. Ruiz-Pérez, and Primitivo Gómez-Cardero
16	Artificial Intelligence in Revision Total Knee Arthroplasty 141
	E. Carlos Rodríguez-Merchán
17	Re-Revision Total Knee Arthroplasty 149
	E. Carlos Rodríguez-Merchán

The Burden of Revision Total Knee Arthroplasty

E. Carlos Rodríguez-Merchán, Hortensia De la Corte-Rodríguez, and Juan M. Román-Belmonte

1.1 Introduction

Total knee arthroplasty (TKA) percentages have risen considerably in the latest decades all around the world [1]. As the amount of TKAs rises, it is feasible to predict the amount of revision TKAs (rTKAs) to increase in parallel [2]. The purpose of this chapter is to analyze the current burdens of rTKA.

1.2 Economic Burden of Hospital Readmissions After Primary TKA

In 2017, Kurtz et al. found that the US rates of 30- and 90-day readmissions after primary TKA (pTKA) were 4% and 7%, respectively [3]. The five most important variables responsible for the cost of 90-day pTKA readmissions were length of stay (LOS), all patient-refined diagnosis-related group (APR DRG) severity, gender, hospital procedure volume, and hospital ownership. After adjusting for covariates, mean 90-day readmission costs reimbursed by private insurance were, on average, US dollars (USD) 1372 greater than Medicare for pTKA. For pTKA, 49% of the total readmission cost in 90 days for the USA was associated with procedure issues, most notably including infections. The conclusion was that hospital readmissions

E. C. Rodríguez-Merchán (✉)
Department of Orthopedic Surgery, La Paz University Hospital, Madrid, Spain

H. De la Corte-Rodríguez
Department of Physical Medicine and Rehabilitation, La Paz University Hospital, Madrid, Spain

J. M. Román-Belmonte
Department of Physical Medicine and Rehabilitation, Cruz Roja San José y Santa Adela University Hospital, Madrid, Spain

© The Author(s), under exclusive license to Springer Nature Switzerland AG 2024
E. C. Rodríguez-Merchán (ed.), *Advances in Revision Total Knee Arthroplasty*,
https://doi.org/10.1007/978-3-031-60445-4_1

up to 90 days after pTKA represented a massive economic burden on the US healthcare system. Approximately half of the total annual economic burden for readmissions in the USA was medical and unrelated to the joint replacement procedure, and half was related to procedural complications. Kutz et al. claimed that additional clinical research was required to determine the extent to which, if any, the LOS during readmissions can be diminished without sacrificing quality or access of care [3].

1.3 Ninety-Day Emergency Department Visits Present a Significant Burden to the Healthcare System

In 2022, Singh et al. analyzed the difference between primary total joint arthroplasty (pTJA) and revision TJA (rTJA) cases in terms of the percentage and reasons associated with 90-day emergency department (ED) visits [4]. Singh et al. retrospectively reviewed all individuals who experienced TJA from 2011 to 2021 at their hospital. Individuals were separated into two groups based on whether they experienced pTJA or rTJA. Overall, 28,033 individuals were included, of whom 24,930 (89%) experienced pTJA and 3103 (11%) experienced rTJA. The overall percentage of 90-day ED visits was substantially lower for individuals who experienced pTJA in comparison to those who experienced rTJA (3.9% versus 7%). Among those who presented to the ED, the readmission percentage was statistically lower for individuals who experienced pTJA compared to rTJA (23.5% versus 32.1%). ED visits presented a substantial burden to the healthcare system. Individuals who experienced rTJA were more likely to present to the ED within 90 days following surgery compared to pTJA individuals. However, among individuals in both groups who visited the ED, 75% did not need readmission [4].

1.4 Projected Economic Burden of Periprosthetic Joint Infection

In 2021, Premkumar et al. analyzed the burden of periprosthetic joint infection (PJI) in the USA. The Nationwide Inpatient Sample (2002–2017) was utilized to recognize rates and associated inpatient costs for pTKA and PJI-related rTKA [5]. Figure 1.1 shows the main results of the study. Although the growth in prevalence

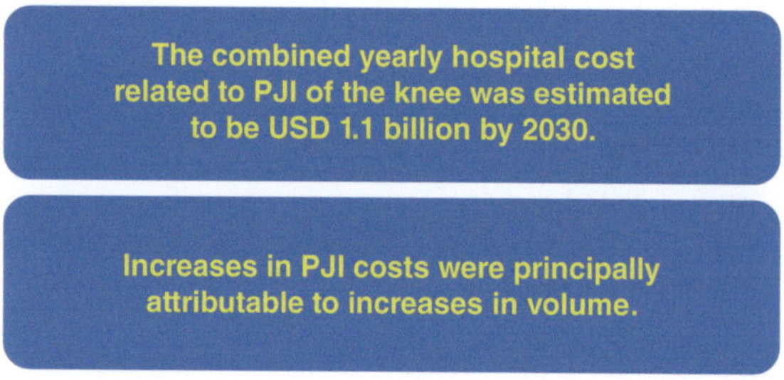

Fig. 1.1 Inpatient costs for primary total knee arthroplasty (TKA) and periprosthetic joint infection (PJI)-related revision TKA: projected economic burden of PJI (Premkumar et al., 2021) [5]. *USD* US dollars

> The combined yearly hospital cost related to PJI of the knee was estimated to be USD 1.1 billion by 2030.

> Increases in PJI costs were principally attributable to increases in volume.

of pTKA had decreased in recent years, the incidence of PJI and the cost per case of PJI endured relatively constant from 2002 to 2017. The conclusion was that there is an urgent need for effective preventive strategies in diminishing rates of PJI after pTKA [5].

1.5 The Economic Impact of Periprosthetic Fractures

In 2022, Crutcher et al. evaluated the economic impact of periprosthetic fractures (PPFs) on a hospital system [6]. Crutcher et al. performed a retrospective study of PPFs of the hip and knee between 2018 and 2019. An analysis of direct inpatient costs was carried out and categorized by a fracture type. Crutcher et al. identified 213 periprosthetic hip and 151 periprosthetic knee fractures. The mean age of hip individuals was 77 years, and 71% were female. The average surgery time was 194 minutes, LOS was 5.01 days, and 71% were discharged to a skilled nursing facility (SNF). The mean age of knee individuals was 76 years, and 79% were female. The average surgery time was 174 min, LOS was 5.12 days, and 70% were discharged to a SNF. The median direct cost of hip fractures was USD 17,108, with Vancouver B2 and B3 costing significantly more at USD 19,987 and USD 23,935, respectively. Figure 1.2 shows the main results of the study. The conclusion was that PPFs created a significant economic impact on hospital systems. Crutcher et al. found that substantially higher costs were associated with injuries needing revision implants [6].

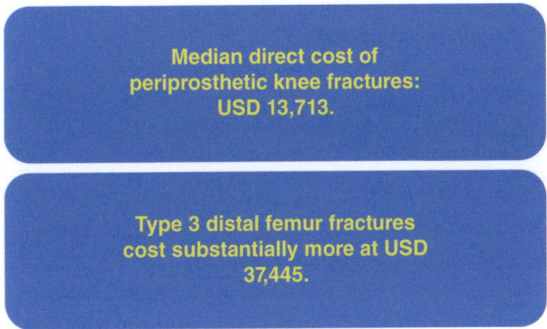

Fig. 1.2 Economic impact of knee periprosthetic fractures (Crutcher et al., 2022) [6]. *USD* US dollars

1.6 The Effect of COVID-19 on Elective TKA Utilization

In a study with level 3 of evidence published in 2022 by Gordon et al., the effect of COVID-19 on elective TKA utilization, patient comorbidity burden, and complications was analyzed [7]. They compared temporal trends in procedural volume, patient demographics, and postoperative adverse events of elective TKA in 2019 and 2020. Utilizing a multicenter, nationwide representative sample, a retrospective query of the 2019–2020 American College of Surgeons National Surgical Quality Improvement Program database was performed for individuals experiencing elective TKA. Temporal trends in utilization, demographics, and LOS were compared pre-COVID-19 (2019 to 2020Q1) with post-COVID-19 (2020Q2 to Q4). Postoperative results were compared by calendar year (2019 versus 2020). A total of 121,415 individuals experienced elective TKA in 2019 ($N = 72,002$) and 2020 ($N = 49,413$), a 31.4% decline. The proportion of hospital-defined "outpatient" TKAs in 2020 was substantially greater than that in 2019 (41.5% versus 25.5%). Elective TKA utilization decreased by 65.1% in 2020Q2 and never returned to pre-pandemic baseline in 2020Q3 to Q4. The average LOS was shorter in 2020 (1.56 versus 1.87 days). The proportion of same-day discharge augmented each quarter from 2019Q1 to Q4 (6.2% to 8.6%) to 2020Q1 to Q4 (8.7% to 17.1%). Total complication percentages were similar in 2019 (4.84%) versus 2020 (4.75%). The 30-day mortality (0.08% versus 0.07%), revision surgery (1% versus 1%), and readmission (2.8% versus 2.6%) percentages were no different between 2019 and 2020. Elective TKA diminished during the second quarter of 2020. A large proportion of surgeries were transitioned to outpatient with percentages of same-day discharge augmenting over the study period, despite no change in adverse events, mortality, and readmission percentages. Patient results were not compromised despite pandemic restrictions for elective surgery [7].

1.7 Thirty-Day Mortality Burden After rTKA

In 2021, Sinclair et al. studied the overall 30-day mortality percentage and the 30-day mortality percentage stratified by age, comorbidity, and septic versus aseptic failure following rTKA [8]. The American College of Surgeons National Surgical Quality Improvement Program was reviewed for all individuals experiencing rTKA from 2011 to 2019. A total of 32,354 individuals who experienced rTKA were identified and categorized as mortality ($N = 115$) or mortality-free ($N = 32,239$). Patient characteristics were compared between groups and further stratified by septic and aseptic failure. The overall 30-day mortality percentage was 0.36%. The percentage of deaths per age cohort (normalized per 1000) is shown in Table 1.1. The rate of deaths per American Society of Anesthesiologists (ASA) class is shown in Table 1.2. Increasing age, greater comorbidity burden, underweight or normal body mass index (BMI), insulin-dependent diabetes, septic revision, and general anesthesia were all related to an augmented risk of mortality after rTKA. Remarkably, 1 in 80

Table 1.1 Thirty-day mortality burden after revision total knee arthroplasty (rTKA): percentage of deaths per age cohort [8]

Cohort (years)	Percentage (%)
18–29	0
30–39	0
40–49	0.18
50–59	0.13
60–69	0.14
70–79	0.40
80–89	1.25
90+	6.93

Table 1.2 Thirty-day mortality burden after revision total knee arthroplasty (rTKA): deaths per ASA (American Society of Anesthesiologists) class [8]

ASA class	Percentage (%)
1	0.30
2	0.06
3	0.39
4	2.41
5	14.29

individuals (1.25%) aged 80–89 years died following rTKA compared to 1 in 720 individuals (0.13%) aged 60–69 years. Individuals who experienced septic revision had a fourfold increase in mortality compared to aseptic revision [8].

1.8 Markup Ratios for pTKA and rTKA Services to Medicare Beneficiaries

In 2023, Rizk et al. affirmed that comprehending markup ratios (MRs), the ratio between a healthcare institution's submitted charge, and the Medicare payment received, for high-volume orthopedic procedures, was mandatory to inform policy about price transparency and diminishing surprise billing [9]. They analyzed the MRs for primary and revision total hip arthroplasty (THA) and TKA services to Medicare beneficiaries between 2013 and 2019 across healthcare settings and geographic regions. A large dataset was queried for all THA and TKA procedures carried out by orthopedic surgeons between 2013 and 2019, utilizing Healthcare Common Procedure Coding System (HCPCS) codes for the most commonly utilized services. Annual MRs, service counts, average submitted charges, average allowed payments, and average Medicare payments were studied. Trends in MRs were evaluated. Rizk et al. assessed 9 THA HCPCS codes, averaging 159,297 procedures a year provided by a mean of 5330 surgeons. They assessed 6 TKA HCPCS codes, averaging 290,244 procedures a year provided by a mean of 7308 surgeons. For knee arthroplasty procedures, a decline was noted for HCPCS code 27438 (patellar arthroplasty with prosthesis) over the study period (8.30–6.62), and HCPCS code 27447 (TKA) had the highest median MR ratio (4.73). For revision knee procedures, the highest median MR was for HCPCS code 27488 (removal of knee prosthesis; 6.12). While no trends were noted for both primary THA and rTHA, median MRs in 2019 for primary hip procedures ranged from 3.83 (hemiarthroplasty) to 5.06 (conversion of previous hip surgery to THA), and HCPCS code 27130 (THA) had a median MR of 4.66. For revision hip procedures, MRs ranged from 3.79 (open treatment of femoral fracture or prosthetic replacement) to 6.10 (revision of THA femoral component). Wisconsin had the highest median MR by state (>9) for primary knee, revision knee, and primary hip procedures. The MRs for primary and revision THA and TKA procedures were strikingly high, as compared to non-orthopedic procedures. These findings represented high levels of excess charges billed, which may pose serious financial burdens to individuals and must be taken into account in future policy discussions to avert price inflation [9].

1.9 Projected Burden of rTKA in Different Countries

1.9.1 China

In 2023, Long et al. investigated the burden and characteristics of rTKA in China [10]. They reviewed 4503 rTKA cases registered in the Hospital Quality Monitoring System in China between 2013 and 2018 utilizing International Classification of Diseases, Ninth Revision, Clinical Modification (ICD-9-CM) codes. Revision burden was calculated by the ratio of the number of revision procedures to the total number of TKA procedures. The rTKA cases accounted for 2.4% of all TKA cases. The revision burden showed an increasing trend from 2013 to 2018 (2.3%–2.5%). Gradual increases in rTKA were found in individuals aged >60 years. The most frequent causes for rTKA were infection (33%) and mechanical failure (19.5%). More than 70% of the individuals were hospitalized in provincial hospitals. A total of 17.6% individuals were hospitalized in a hospital outside the province of their residence. The hospitalization charges continued to augment between 2013 and 2015 and remained roughly stable over the next 3 years. There was a growing trend of revision burden during the study period. The focalized nature of operations in a few higher volume regions was found, and many individuals had to travel to obtain their rTKA [10].

1.9.2 Germany

In a study with level 3 of evidence published by Klug et al. in 2021, they provided an overview of treatment changes during the last decade and projected the expected burden of pTKA and rTKA for the next 30 years [1]. Comprehensive nationwide data from Germany was utilized to quantify pTKA and rTKA percentages as a function of age and gender. Projections were carried out with utilization of a Poisson regression models and a combination of exponential smoothing and autoregressive integrated moving average models on historical procedure percentages in relation to official population projections from 2020 to 2050. The prevalence rate of pTKAs was projected to augment by about 43% to 299 per 100,000 inhabitants, leading to a projected total number of 225,957 pTKAs in 2050. This increase has been related to a growing number of TKA carried out in male individuals, with the highest increase modelled in individuals between 50 and 65 years of age. At the same time, the yearly total number of revision procedures was forecast to augment even more quickly by almost 90%, accounting for 47,313 procedures by 2050. Those numbers were primarily associated with a rising number of rTKAs secondary to PJI. Utilizing this country-specific forecast approach, a rising number of pTKA and an even more quickly growing number of rTKA, especially for PJI, was projected until 2050, which will inevitably provide a huge challenge for the future healthcare system [1].

1.9.3 Southern Korea

In 2021, Kim et al. published a study (level 3 of evidence) aimed to document the TKA utilization in Korea from 2010 to 2018, to assess whether rapid increase in TKA utilization had been maintained, and to calculate the projected TKA burden to 2030 based on the current utilization [11]. Using the Health Insurance Review and Assessment Korean database, procedural percentage, growth percentage, and revision burden of pTKAs and rTKAs in Southern Korea between 2010 and 2018 were analyzed. Kim et al. observed that between 2010 and 2018, procedural rate of primary and rTKAs has augmented by 35% and 68%, respectively. More than 85% of primary and rTKAs were carried out on female individuals, and the subgroup of individuals aged ≥80 years showed a marked increase in pTKA and rTKA use. The number of pTKAs and rTKAs was predicted to increase between 53% and 91% and between 75% and 155%, respectively, by 2030. The conclusion was that between 2010 and 2018, the procedural percentages of pTKAs and rTKAs in Southern Korea augmented gradually by 35% and 68%, respectively, and previously found striking growth percentage had markedly slowed. Nonetheless, compared to 2018, the burdens of pTKAs and rTKAs were projected to increase up to 91% and 155%, respectively, by 2030 [11].

1.9.4 United States

In 2023, Livshetz et al. investigated the prevalence of rTKA; patient and hospital characteristics; adverse events, hospital LOSs, and discharge dispositions; and costs, charges, and payer types [2]. All individuals who experienced rTKA between 2009 and 2016 were identified from the National Inpatient Sample database utilizing International Classification of Diseases, Ninth Revision and Tenth Revision codes and were studied. Over our study period, there was a 4.3% decrease in the prevalence of rTKA. The mean age of individuals who experienced rTKA was 65 years, and a majority were female (58%). Mean hospital LOS diminished from 4.1 days in 2009 to 3.3 days in 2016. The percentage of several adverse events

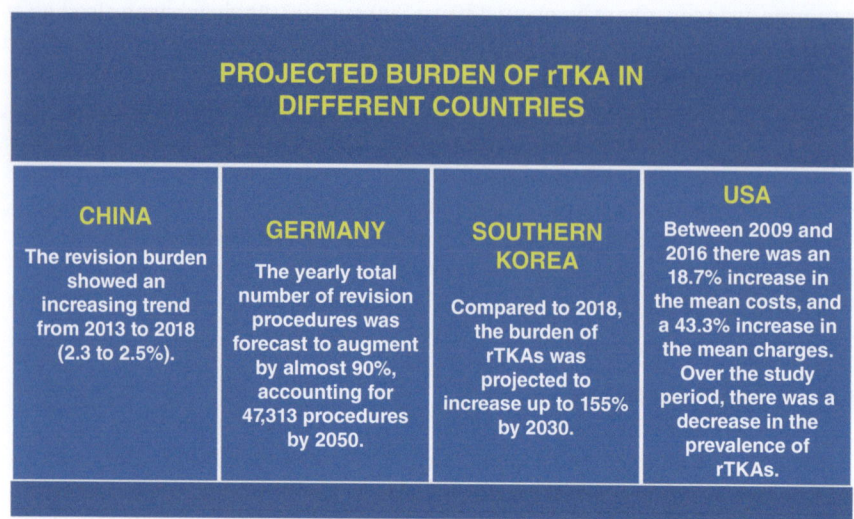

Fig. 1.3 Main data on the projected burden of revision total knee arthroplasty (rTKA) in different countries [1, 2, 10, 11]

diminished substantially over our study period including myocardial infarction, cardiac arrest, transfusion, pneumonia, urinary tract infection, and mortality. A substantially lower rate of rTKA individuals were discharged to a skilled nursing facility in 2016 (26.5%) compared with 2009 (31.6%). There was an 18.7% increase in the mean costs and a 43.3% increase in the mean charges. Over the study period, there was a decrease in the prevalence of rTKAs. In spite of potential improvements in pTKA, the burden associated with rTKA remains large [2]. Figure 1.3 summarizes the main data on the projected burden of rTKA in different countries.

1.10 Conclusions

TKA rates have augmented considerably in the recent decades all around the world. As the amount of TKAs rises, it is plausible to forecast the amount of rTKAs to increase in parallel. In this chapter, the main burdens of rTKA have been analyzed. The reported 30-day mortality rate after rTKA is noteworthy: 0.36% on average. Regarding the percentage of deaths per age, 1.25% of individuals aged 80–89 years die following rTKA compared to 0.13% of individuals aged 60–69 years. Besides, individuals who experience septic revision had a fourfold increase in mortality compared to aseptic revision. In a study, rTKAs were projected to increase up to 155% by 2030. In the other study, the yearly total number of rTKAs was forecast to augment by almost 90% by 2050. In short, the burden associated with rTKA remains large.

References

1. Klug A, Gramlich Y, Rudert M, Drees P, Hoffmann R, Weißenberger M, et al. The projected volume of primary and revision total knee arthroplasty will place an immense burden on future health care systems over the next 30 years. Knee Surg Sports Traumatol Arthrosc. 2021;29(10):3287–98. https://doi.org/10.1007/s00167-020-06154-7.
2. Livshetz I, Sussman BH, Papas V, Mohamed NS, Salem HS, Delanois RE, et al. Analyzing the burden of revision total knee arthroplasty in the United States between 2009 and 2016. J Knee Surg. 2023;36(2):121–31. https://doi.org/10.1055/s-0041-1731324.
3. Kurtz SM, Lau EC, Ong KL, Adler EM, Kolisek FR, Manley MT. Which clinical and patient factors influence the national economic burden of hospital readmissions after total joint arthroplasty? Clin Orthop Relat Res. 2017;475(12):2926–37. https://doi.org/10.1007/s11999-017-5244-6.
4. Singh V, Anil U, Kurapatti M, Robin JX, Schwarzkopf R, Rozell JC. Emergency department visits following total joint arthroplasty: do revisions present a higher burden? Bone Jt Open. 2022;3(7):543–8. https://doi.org/10.1302/2633-1462.37.BJO-2022-0026.R1.
5. Premkumar A, Kolin DA, Farley KX, Wilson JM, McLawhorn AS, Cross MB, et al. Projected economic burden of periprosthetic joint infection of the hip and knee in the United States. J Arthroplast. 2021;36(5):1484–1489.e3. https://doi.org/10.1016/j.arth.2020.12.005.
6. Crutcher JP Jr, Tompkins G, Rollier G, Sypher K, Valderrama R, Duwelius PJ. The economic impact of lower extremity periprosthetic fractures in a large hospital system. J Arthroplast. 2022;37(7S):S439–43. https://doi.org/10.1016/j.arth.2022.03.012.
7. Gordon AM, Magruder ML, Conway CA, Sheth BK, Erez O. The effect of COVID-19 on elective total knee arthroplasty utilization, patient comorbidity burden, and complications in the United States: a nationwide analysis. J Am Acad Orthop Surg. 2022;30(24):e1599–611. https://doi.org/10.5435/JAAOS-D-22-00193.
8. Sinclair ST, Orr MN, Rothfusz CA, Klika AK, McLaughlin JP, Piuzzi NS. Understanding the 30-day mortality burden after revision total knee arthroplasty. Arthroplast Today. 2021;11:205–11. https://doi.org/10.1016/j.artd.2021.08.019.
9. Rizk AA, Kim AG, Bernhard Z, Moyal A, Acuña AJ, Hecht CJ 2nd, et al. Mark-up trends in contemporary Medicare primary and revision total joint arthroplasty. J Arthroplast. 2023;38(9):1642–51. https://doi.org/10.1016/j.arth.2023.03.058.
10. Long H, Xie D, Zeng C, Wang H, Lei G, Yang T. Burden and characteristics of revision total knee arthroplasty in China: a national study based on hospitalized cases. J Arthroplast. 2023;38(7):1320–1325.e2. https://doi.org/10.1016/j.arth.2023.02.052.
11. Kim TW, Kang SB, Chang CB, Moon SY, Lee YK, Koo KH. Current trends and projected burden of primary and revision total knee arthroplasty in Korea between 2010 and 2030. J Arthroplast. 2021;36(1):93–101. https://doi.org/10.1016/j.arth.2020.06.064.

The Impact of Tobacco Use on Revision Total Knee Arthroplasty Outcomes

2

E. Carlos Rodríguez-Merchán, Hortensia De la Corte-Rodríguez, and Juan M. Román-Belmonte

2.1 Introduction

In 2019, Matharu et al. reported that smoking was associated with more medical adverse events, higher analgesia employment, and augmented mortality following total knee arthroplasty (TKA). Most adverse results were diminished in ex-smokers; consequently, smoking cessation should be encouraged prior to TKA [1].

In 2022, Rajaee et al. affirmed that smoking was frequent among individuals experiencing elective TKA, and its prevalence continues to increase. Smoking was associated with higher hospital costs as well as higher percentages of immediate inpatient adverse events [2]. In 2022, Simmons et al. reported that nearly 1 in 10 individuals experiencing elective TKA continued to smoke and maintained a higher risk of postoperative adverse events [3]. Tobacco use has been related to an augmented risk of periprosthetic joint infection (PJI) [4].

In a systematic review published in 2022, Yue et al. affirmed that smoking individuals experiencing TKA are at augmented risk of many adverse events, inpatient mortality, persistent opioid consumption, and worse 1-year patient-reported outcomes (PROMs). Presurgical protocols for these results should give special consideration to smoking individuals [5].

E. C. Rodríguez-Merchán (✉)
Department of Orthopedic Surgery, La Paz University Hospital, Madrid, Spain

H. De la Corte-Rodríguez
Department of Physical Medicine and Rehabilitation, La Paz University Hospital, Madrid, Spain

J. M. Román-Belmonte
Department of Physical Medicine and Rehabilitation, Cruz Roja San José y Santa Adela University Hospital, Madrid, Spain

© The Author(s), under exclusive license to Springer Nature Switzerland AG 2024
E. C. Rodríguez-Merchán (ed.), *Advances in Revision Total Knee Arthroplasty*, https://doi.org/10.1007/978-3-031-60445-4_2

In a study with level 3 of evidence published in 2023 by Waters et al., it was observed that smokeless tobacco usage was associated with higher percentages of both medical and joint adverse events after primary TKA (pTKA). However, smoking was associated with higher risk for adverse events than smokeless tobacco usage [6]. In 2023, Starzer et al. stated that current smoking raises risk of soft-tissue adverse events and revision after pTKA, especially due to hematoma and restricted movement. Smoking cessation programs could diminish the risk of revision surgery [7].

The purpose of this chapter is to analyze the impact of tobacco use on revision TKA (rTKA).

2.2 Current Tobacco Use Is Associated with Higher Percentages of Implant Revision Following Primary Total Knee Arthroplasty

According to Singh et al., tobacco smoking is a risk factor for various adverse postoperative results [8]. In 2015, they compared the percentages of adverse events in current tobacco users and nonusers who experienced primary total hip arthroplasty (pTHA) or pTKA. All individuals who experienced pTHA or pTKA at the Mayo Clinic from 2010 to 2013 were included in the study. Current tobacco usage was defined as the use of cigarettes, cigars, pipes, or smokeless tobacco reported at the time of index THA or TKA; current nonusers were former users or never users. Tobacco usage status was accessible for 7926 individuals (95%) and not accessible for 446 individuals (5%); 565 (7%) were current tobacco users. Compared to nonusers, current tobacco users were more likely to be male and less likely to be obese and to be older than 60 years and have Charlson score >0 or have experienced pTKA rather than pTHA. The hazard ratios for periprosthetic joint infection (PJI) were higher in current tobacco users than in nonusers. No substantial differences were found for periprosthetic fractures or superficial infections. Sing et al. observed that current tobacco usage was associated with high risk of PJI and implant revision after pTHA or pTKA. They concluded that future research should determine the optimal time for tobacco use cessation prior to elective pTHA and pTKA to ameliorate short-run and long-run arthroplasty results [8].

2.3 Smoking Is Associated with Earlier Time to Revision Total Knee Arthroplasty

In 2017, Lim et al. stated that smoking was associated with early postoperative adverse events, increased length of hospital stay, and an increased risk of revision after TKA [9]. However, the impact of smoking on time to revision TKA was not known. In the study, a total of 619 pTKAs referred to an academic tertiary center for rTKA were retrospectively stratified according to the individual smoking status.

Fig. 2.1 Risks of early revision total knee arthroplasty (rTKA) in smokers, nonsmokers, and ex-smokers [9]

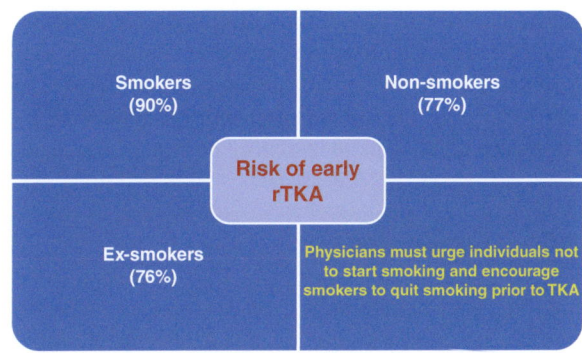

Smoking status was then analyzed for associations with time to rTKA. The association was also analyzed according to the indication for rTKA. Smokers (37/41, 90%) have an increased risk of earlier revision for any reason compared to nonsmokers (274/357, 77%). Smokers (37/41, 90%) have an increased risk of earlier revision for any reason compared to ex-smokers (168/221, 76%). Subgroup analysis did not show a difference in indication for rTKA. Smokers were at increased risk of earlier rTKA when compared to nonsmokers and ex-smokers. The risk for ex-smokers was similar to that of nonsmokers. Smoking seemed to have an all-or-none impact on earlier rTKA as individuals who smoked more did not have higher risk of early rTKA. The outcomes of this study highlighted the need for physicians to urge individuals not to begin smoking and encourage smokers to quit smoking before pTKA [9] (Fig. 2.1).

2.4 Tobacco Use Is Associated with more Severe Adverse Results than Morbid Obesity Following Aseptic rTKA

According to Hagerty et al., the association of morbid obesity with augmented rTKA adverse events is potentially confounded by concurrent risk factors [10]. In 2023, Hagerty et al. assessed whether morbid obesity was more strongly associated with adverse aseptic rTKA results than diabetes or tobacco use history when present as a solitary major risk factor. Demographic characteristics, surgical indications, and adverse results (reoperation, revision, infection, and amputation) were compared between 270 index aseptic rTKA carried out for individuals with morbid obesity ($N = 73$), diabetes ($N = 72$), or tobacco use ($N = 125$) and 239 "healthy" controls without these risk factors at a mean 75.7 months. There was no difference in 2-year reoperation percentage (17.8 versus 17.6%) or component revision percentage (8.2 versus 8.4%) between morbidly obese and healthy individuals. However, higher reoperation percentages were found in individuals with diabetes and tobacco use history, including higher infection and above knee amputation percentages in individuals with tobacco use history. An independent association between smoking history and amputation risk was found. Morbid obesity was not associated with an augmented risk of reoperation or component revision compared with healthy individuals experiencing aseptic revision. Following aseptic rTKA, tobacco use was associated with augmented reoperation and above knee amputation. Hagerty et al. concluded that further research will be helpful to ascertain whether risk decline efforts are efficacious in lessening postoperative adverse events risks [10].

2.5 Conclusions

Smoking is associated with early postoperative adverse events, augmented length of hospital stay, and an augmented risk of revision after TKA. Smokers have an augmented risk of earlier revision for any cause compared to nonsmokers. Smokers have an augmented risk of earlier revision for any cause compared to ex-smokers. Smokers are at augmented risk of earlier rTKA when compared to nonsmokers and ex-smokers. The risk for ex-smokers is similar to that of nonsmokers. Smoking seems to have an all-or-none influence on earlier rTKA as individuals who smoke more do not have higher risk of early rTKA. Physicians must recommend individuals not to commence smoking and urge smokers to cease smoking prior to pTKA.

References

1. Matharu GS, Mouchti S, Twigg S, Delmestri A, Murray DW, Judge A, et al. The effect of smoking on outcomes following primary total hip and knee arthroplasty: a population-based cohort study of 117,024 patients. Acta Orthop. 2019;90(6):559–67. https://doi.org/10.1080/17453674.2019.1649510.
2. Rajaee SS, Debbi EM, Paiement GD, Spitzer AI. Increased prevalence, complications, and costs of smokers undergoing total knee arthroplasty. J Knee Surg. 2022;35(1):91–5. https://doi.org/10.1055/s-0040-1713128.
3. Simmons HL, Grits D, Orr M, Murray T, Klika AK, Piuzzi NS. Trends in the prevalence and postoperative surgical complications for smokers who underwent a total knee arthroplasty from 2011 to 2019: an analysis of 406,553 patients. J Knee Surg. 2023;36(9):957–64. https://doi.org/10.1055/s-0042-1748819.
4. Rodriguez-Merchan EC, Delgado-Martinez AD. Risk factors for periprosthetic joint infection after primary total knee arthroplasty. J Clin Med. 2022;11(20):6128. https://doi.org/10.3390/jcm11206128.
5. Yue C, Cui G, Ma M, Tang Y, Li H, Liu Y, et al. Associations between smoking and clinical outcomes after total hip and knee arthroplasty: a systematic review and meta-analysis. Front Surg. 2022;9:970537. https://doi.org/10.3389/fsurg.2022.970537.
6. Waters TL, Collins LK, Cole MW, Salas Z, Springer BD, Sherman WF. Smokeless tobacco use is associated with worse outcomes following total knee arthroplasty. J Arthroplast. 2023;38(7):1281–6. https://doi.org/10.1016/j.arth.2023.01.035.
7. Starzer M, Smolle MA, Vielgut I, Hauer G, Leitner L, Radl R, et al. Smokers have increased risk of soft-tissue complications following primary elective TKA. Arch Orthop Trauma Surg. 2023;143(8):4689–95. https://doi.org/10.1007/s00402-023-04771-8.
8. Singh JA, Schleck C, Harmsen WS, Jacob AK, Warner DO, Lewallen DG. Current tobacco use is associated with higher rates of implant revision and deep infection after total hip or knee arthroplasty: a prospective cohort study. BMC Med. 2015;13:283. https://doi.org/10.1186/s12916-015-0523-0.

9. Lim CT, Goodman SB, Huddleston JI 3rd, Harris AHS, Bhowmick S, Maloney WJ, et al. Smoking is associated with earlier time to revision of total knee arthroplasty. Knee. 2017;24(5):1182–6. https://doi.org/10.1016/j.knee.2017.05.014.
10. Hagerty MP, Walker-Santiago R, Tegethoff JD, Stronach BM, Keeney JA. Tobacco use is associated with more severe adverse outcomes than morbid obesity after aseptic revision TKA. J Knee Surg. 2023;36(2):201–7. https://doi.org/10.1055/s-0041-1731459.

The Impact of Obesity on Revision Total Knee Arthroplasty Outcomes

3

E. Carlos Rodríguez-Merchán, Hortensia De la Corte-Rodríguez, and Juan M. Román-Belmonte

3.1 Introduction

There is a large body of literature on the impact of obesity [body mass index (BMI), 30–39.9 kg/m^2] on primary total knee arthroplasty (pTKA) outcomes, some of which (those considered to be of most interest) are briefly discussed below [1–14]. However, there are few publications on the impact of obesity on the outcomes of revision total knee arthroplasty (rTKA).

In a study published in 2019, an increased mid- to long-run revision rate after pTKA in morbidly obese individuals was encountered; however, these individuals had a functional recovery which was similar to nonobese individuals. There was also an increased risk of perioperative adverse events, such as superficial wound infection [1].

In another publication, morbid obesity (BMI ≥40 kg/m^2) seemed to be independently associated with a higher risk for a small number of select in-hospital postoperative adverse events and mortality. However, the independent influence of morbid obesity seemed to be fairly modest, and morbid obesity did not appear to be an independent risk factor for many systemic adverse events [2].

E. C. Rodríguez-Merchán (✉)
Department of Orthopedic Surgery, La Paz University Hospital, Madrid, Spain

H. De la Corte-Rodríguez
Department of Physical Medicine and Rehabilitation, La Paz University Hospital, Madrid, Spain

J. M. Román-Belmonte
Department of Physical Medicine and Rehabilitation, Cruz Roja San José y Santa Adela University Hospital, Madrid, Spain

© The Author(s), under exclusive license to Springer Nature Switzerland AG 2024
E. C. Rodríguez-Merchán (ed.), *Advances in Revision Total Knee Arthroplasty*, https://doi.org/10.1007/978-3-031-60445-4_3

In 2022, it was reported that the gained benefit in functional result surpassed the increase in risk of revision and adverse events for the morbidly obese in pTKA [3].

According to King et al., cementless TKA utilizing a highly porous tibial baseplate in morbidly obese individuals showed excellent clinical outcomes with 98% survivorship at 5 years and seemed to offer durable long-run biologic fixation as an alternative to mechanical cement fixation in this group of individuals [4].

Aggarwal et al. found that results of pTKA were not definitively worse in obese individuals when compared to matched nonobese individuals [5].

In 2022, Yan et al. stated that bariatric surgery before pTKA may raise the risk of perioperative blood transfusion and also the risk of revision and infection in long-run follow-up [6].

Sinicrope et al. found that morbidly obese individuals had a higher failure due to aseptic loosening with cemented TKA with decreasing survivorship over time. The utilization of cementless TKA in morbidly obese individuals with the potential of durable long-run biologic fixation and increased survivorship seemed to be a promising alternative to mechanical cement fixation [7].

In 2022, Goh et al. reported that obese patients with BMI ≥ 35 kg/m^2 experiencing cementless and cemented pTKA of the same modern design had comparable results and survivorship at early to mid-run follow-up [8]. Kim et al. reported that weight gain postoperatively was associated with inferior results. Substantial weight loss before surgery led to a "rebound" in weight gain and independently augmented risk for all-cause revision [9]. According to Rassir et al., obesity seemed to be associated with some short-run revision risks after pTKA but was not associated with an overall increase in revision rate [10]. Onggo et al. affirmed that obesity is a substantial, modifiable risk factor for increased adverse events after pTKA [11].

In a study with level 3 of evidence published in 2022 Wall et al., the rates of all-cause revision and revision for infection, loosening, instability, and pain were compared for nonobese individuals (BMI, 18.50–29.99 kg/m^2), class I and II obese patients (BMI, 30–39.99 kg/m^2), and class III obese patients (BMI, ≥ 40 kg/m^2). The reasons for the procedures included infection in 39.7%, loosening in 14.8%, instability in 12%, and pain in 6.1%. Class I and II obese individuals had a higher risk of all-cause revision and revision for infection than nonobese individuals. Class III obese individuals had a higher risk of all-cause revision after 1 year, revision for infection after 3 months, and revision for loosening than nonobese individuals. The risks of revision for instability and pain were comparable among cohorts [12].

According to Hagerty et al., morbid obesity was not associated with an increased risk of reoperation or component revision compared with healthy individuals experiencing aseptic revision [13]. The sequence of surgery in individuals experiencing both bariatric surgery and pTKA did not seem to be associated with weight loss after bariatric surgery or the risk of revision after pTKA [14].

The purpose of this chapter is to review the most recent publications concerning the impact of obesity on rTKA.

3.2 Obesity Trends in rTKA

In 2016, Odum et al. stated that the utilization of pTKA in obese individuals had increased substantially over the past decade in spite of overwhelming information that suggested higher failure rates. As such, it was reasonable to expect a parallel increase in obesity rates among rTKA individuals. Adum et al. analyzed longitudinal trends in obesity rates among rTKA individuals [15]. They identified 451,982 rTKA individuals utilizing 2002–2012 Nationwide Inpatient Sample weighted discharge data. The Agency for Healthcare Research and Quality obesity comorbidity indicator was utilized to identify 70,470 obese individuals (BMI >30) and 335,257 nonobese individuals. The obesity rate among rTKA individuals increased substantially from 9.74% in 2002 to 24.57% in 2012. Individuals treated in 2011 or 2012 were over four times as likely to be obese, compared to individuals treated in 2002. Other independent factors that were substantially associated with higher obesity percentages include female individuals and individuals between the ages of 45 and 64 years. The more than fourfold increase in the obesity rate among individuals experiencing rTKA, particularly the middle-age group, over the 2002–2012 decade was an alarming trend [15].

3.3 Early Complications of rTKA in Morbidly Obese Individuals

A retrospective cohort study was published by Carter et al. to investigate the early adverse events of rTKA in morbidly obese individuals. Revision TKA procedures were carried out between January 2009 and December 2012 at a single center. Comparisons were made between individuals with a normal BMI (18.5–25) and individuals with morbid obesity (BMI >40). Thirty-three of 141 morbidly obese individuals (23.4%) had an adverse event compared to 10 of 96 individuals with a BMI 18.5–25 (10.4%). Morbidly obese individuals were younger (69.3 vs. 61.4 years), and their most common adverse event in comparison with individuals with normal BMI was wound healing problems. Morbidly obese individuals were at a substantially increased percentage of early adverse events after rTKA compared to a normal weight group, especially with regard to wound complications. The morbidly obese cohort was substantially younger at the time of rTKA [16].

3.4 The Effects of Obesity with rTKAs

In a study with level 3 of evidence, Watts et al. analyzed whether individuals with morbid obesity were at greater risk for repeat revision, reoperation, or periprosthetic joint infection (PJI) compared with individuals without obesity (BMI <30 kg/m^2) after a rTKA carried out for aseptic reasons and whether individuals who are not

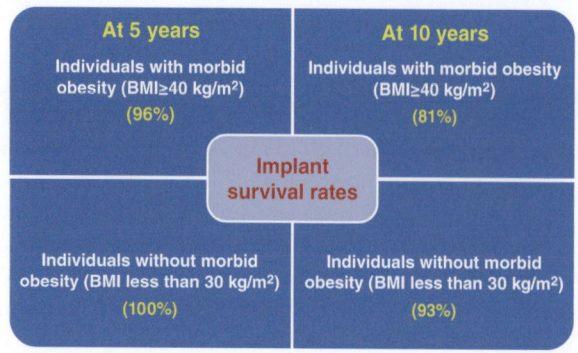

Fig. 3.1 Implant survival rates in patients with morbid obesity versus patients without morbid obesity at 5 and 10 years [17]. BMI = body mass index

obese accomplished higher Knee Society pain and function scores after rTKA for aseptic reasons [17]. They utilized a retrospective cohort study with 1:1 matching for sex, age (±3 years), and date of surgery (±1 year) to compare individuals with morbid obesity with individuals without obesity with respect to repeat revision, reoperation, and PJI. They analyzed 1291 index both-component (femoral and tibial) aseptic rTKAs carried out during a 15-year period (1992–2007). Of these, 120 revisions were in individuals with morbid obesity and 624 were in individuals with a BMI less than 30 kg/m². Watts et al. then considered only individuals with a minimum 5-year follow-up, which was available for 77% of individuals with morbid obesity and 76% of individuals with a BMI less than 30 kg/m². All individuals with morbid obesity who met criteria were included (morbid obesity cohort, $N = 93$; average follow-up, 7.9 years) and compared with a matched group of individuals with a BMI less than 30 kg/m² (non-morbid obesity cohort, $N = 93$; average follow-up, 7.3 years). Overall, individuals with morbid obesity had an increased risk of repeat revision, reoperation, and PJI. Implant survival rates are shown in Fig. 3.1. At 10 years, The Knee Society pain (90) and function (61) scores were higher in individuals with a BMI less than 30 kg/m² compared with individuals with morbid obesity. Morbid obesity was associated with increased percentages of re-revision, reoperation, and PJI following aseptic rTKA [17].

3.5 Outcomes of rTKA in Obese and Morbidly Obese Individuals

In 2023, Bigham et al. investigated the role of BMI in the cause for rTKA and whether BMI classification was predictive of results. A multi-institutional database was generated, including rTKAs from 2012 to 2019. Individuals were compared utilizing three BMI categories: nonobese (18.5–29.9), obese (30–39.9), and morbidly obese. Figure 3.2 summarizes the results of this study [18].

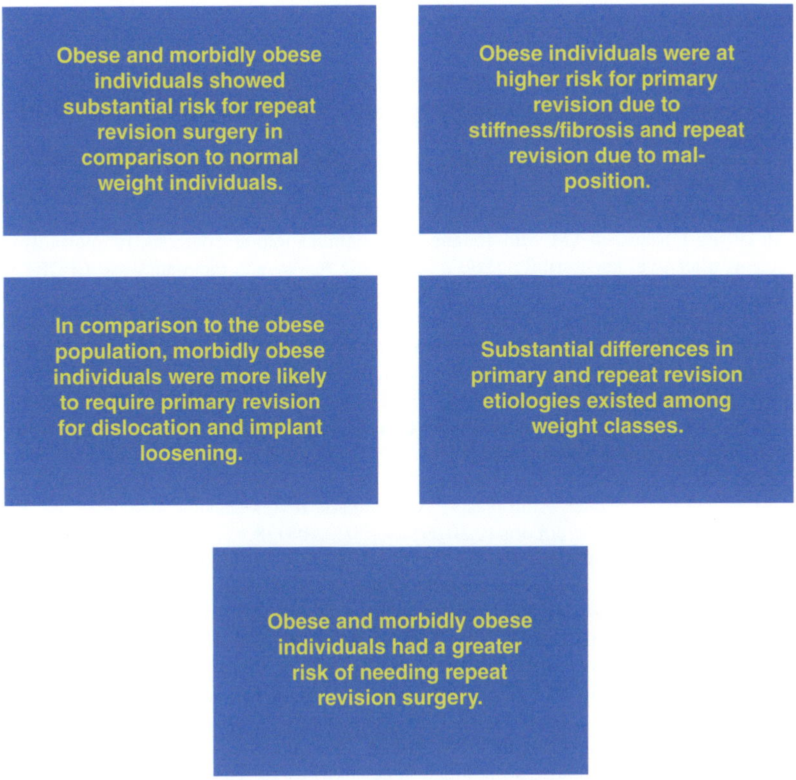

> **Obese and morbidly obese individuals showed substantial risk for repeat revision surgery in comparison to normal weight individuals.**

> **Obese individuals were at higher risk for primary revision due to stiffness/fibrosis and repeat revision due to malposition.**

> **In comparison to the obese population, morbidly obese individuals were more likely to require primary revision for dislocation and implant loosening.**

> **Substantial differences in primary and repeat revision etiologies existed among weight classes.**

> **Obese and morbidly obese individuals had a greater risk of needing repeat revision surgery.**

Fig. 3.2 Individuals were compared utilizing three body mass index (BMI) categories: nonobese (18.5–29.9 kg/m^2), obese (30–39.9 kg/m^2), and morbidly obese (≥40 kg/m^2) [18]

3.6 Conclusions

A study published in 2015 found that patients with morbid obesity had an increased risk of repeat revision, reoperation, and PJI than patients without obesity. Implant survival rates were 96% and 100% at 5 years and 81% and 93% at 10 years for the patients with morbid obesity and those without morbid obesity, respectively.

In 2023, individuals were compared utilizing three BMI categories: nonobese (18.5–29.9 kg/m^2), obese (30–39.9 kg/m^2), and morbidly obese (≥40 kg/m^2). Obese and morbidly obese individuals exhibited substantial risk for repeat revision surgery in comparison to normal weight individuals. Obese individuals were at higher risk for primary revision due to stiffness and repeat revision due to malposition. In comparison to the obese population, morbidly obese individuals were more likely to need primary revision for dislocation and implant loosening. Substantial differences in primary and repeat revision etiologies were encountered among weight classes. Moreover, obese and morbidly obese individuals have a greater risk of needing repeat revision surgery.

References

1. Boyce L, Prasad A, Barrett M, Dawson-Bowling S, Millington S, Hanna SA, et al. The outcomes of total knee arthroplasty in morbidly obese patients: a systematic review of the literature. Arch Orthop Trauma Surg. 2019;139(4):553–60. https://doi.org/10.1007/s00402-019-03127-5.
2. D'Apuzzo MR, Novicoff WM, Browne JA. The John Insall award: morbid obesity independently impacts complications, mortality, and resource use after TKA. Clin Orthop Relat Res. 2015;473(1):57–63. https://doi.org/10.1007/s11999-014-3668-9.
3. van Tilburg J, Rathsach AM. Mid- to long-term complications and outcome for morbidly obese patients after total knee arthroplasty: a systematic review and meta-analysis. EFORT Open Rev. 2022;7(5):295–304. https://doi.org/10.1530/EOR-21-0090.
4. King BA, Miller AJ, Nadar AC, Smith LS, Yakkanti MR, Harwin SF, et al. Cementless total knee arthroplasty using a highly porous tibial baseplate in morbidly obese patients: minimum 5-year follow-up. J Knee Surg. 2023;36(9):995–1000. https://doi.org/10.1055/s-0042-1748900.
5. Aggarwal VA, Sambandam SN, Wukich DK. The impact of obesity on total knee arthroplasty outcomes: a retrospective matched cohort study. J Clin Orthop Trauma. 2022;33:101987. https://doi.org/10.1016/j.jcot.2022.101987.
6. Yan M, Zheng G, Long Z, Pan Q, Wang X, Li Y, et al. Does bariatric surgery really benefit patients before total knee arthroplasty? A systematic review and meta-analysis. Int J Surg. 2022;104:106778. https://doi.org/10.1016/j.ijsu.2022.106778.
7. Sinicrope BJ, Feher AW, Bhimani SJ, Smith LS, Harwin SF, Yakkanti MR, et al. Increased survivorship of cementless versus cemented TKA in the morbidly obese. A minimum 5-year follow-up. J Arthroplast. 2019;34(2):309–14. https://doi.org/10.1016/j.arth.2018.10.016.
8. Goh GS, Fillingham YA, Sutton RM, Small I, Courtney PM, Hozack WJ. Cemented versus cementless total knee arthroplasty in obese patients with body mass index ≥ 35 kg/m^2: a contemporary analysis of 812 patients. J Arthroplast. 2022;37(4):688–693.e1. https://doi.org/10.1016/j.arth.2021.12.038.
9. Kim BI, Cochrane NH, O'Donnell JA, Wu M, Wellman SS, Ryan S, et al. Preoperative weight loss and postoperative weight gain independently increase risk for revision after primary total knee arthroplasty. J Arthroplast. 2022;37(4):674–82. https://doi.org/10.1016/j.arth.2021.12.003.
10. Rassir R, Sierevelt IN, van Steenbergen LN, Nolte PA. Is obesity associated with short-term revision after total knee arthroplasty? An analysis of 121,819 primary procedures from the Dutch Arthroplasty Register. Knee. 2020;27(6):1899–906. https://doi.org/10.1016/j.knee.2020.09.020.
11. Onggo JR, Ang JJM, Onggo JD, de Steiger R, Hau R. Greater risk of all-cause revisions and complications for obese patients in 3 106 381 total knee arthroplasties: a meta-analysis and systematic review. ANZ J Surg. 2021;91(11):2308–21. https://doi.org/10.1111/ans.17138.
12. Wall CJ, Vertullo CJ, Kondalsamy-Chennakesavan S, Lorimer MF, de Steiger RN. A prospective, longitudinal study of the influence of obesity on total knee arthroplasty revision rate: results from the Australian Orthopaedic Association National Joint Replacement Registry. J Bone Joint Surg Am. 2022;104(15):1386–92. https://doi.org/10.2106/JBJS.21.01491.
13. Hagerty MP, Walker-Santiago R, Tegethoff JD, Stronach BM, Keeney JA. Tobacco use is associated with more severe adverse outcomes than morbid obesity after aseptic revision TKA. J Knee Surg. 2023;36(2):201–7. https://doi.org/10.1055/s-0041-1731459.
14. Ighani Arani P, Wretenberg P, Stenberg E, Ottosson J, W-Dahl A. Total knee arthroplasty and bariatric surgery: change in BMI and risk of revision depending on sequence of surgery. BMC Surg. 2023;23(1):53 https://doi.org/10.1186/s12893-023-01951-6.
15. Odum SM, Van Doren BA, Springer BD. National obesity trends in revision total knee arthroplasty. J Arthroplast. 2016;31(9 Suppl):136–9. https://doi.org/10.1016/j.arth.2015.12.055.
16. Carter J, Springer B, Curtin BM. Early complications of revision total knee arthroplasty in morbidly obese patients. Eur J Orthop Surg Traumatol. 2019;29(5):1101–4. https://doi.org/10.1007/s00590-019-02403-9.

17. Watts CD, Wagner ER, Houdek MT, Lewallen DG, Mabry TM. Morbid obesity: increased risk of failure after aseptic revision TKA. Clin Orthop Relat Res. 2015;473(8):2621–7. https://doi.org/10.1007/s11999-015-4283-0.
18. Bigham WR, Lensing G, Walters M, Bhanat E, Keeney J, Stronach BM. Outcomes of total knee arthroplasty revisions in obese and morbidly obese patient populations. J Arthroplast. 2023;38(9):1822–6. https://doi.org/10.1016/j.arth.2023.03.017.

Impact of Preoperative Opioid Use on Revision Total Knee Arthroplasty Outcomes

E. Carlos Rodríguez-Merchán

4.1 Introduction

In 2017, Rozell et al. stated that multimodal pain protocols had diminished opioid requirements and reduced adverse events after elective primary total hip arthroplasty (pTHA) and primary total knee arthroplasty (pTKA) [1]. However, these protocols were not universally effective. That is why they studied the risk factors related to augmented opioid requirements and the impact of preoperative narcotic use on the length of stay (LOS) and in-hospital adverse events following pTHA or pTKA. Rozell et al. prospectively assessed a consecutive series of 802 individuals experiencing elective pTHA and pTKA over a 9-month period. All individuals were treated utilizing a multimodal pain protocol. Of the 802 individuals, 266 (33%) needed intravenous narcotic rescue. Individuals aged <75 years and with preoperative narcotic utilization were more likely to need rescue. It was shown that preoperative narcotic utilization was the largest independent predictor of augmented postoperative opioid requirements. These individuals developed more in-hospital adverse events. This was associated with an increased LOS and a 2.5-times risk of needing oral narcotics at 3 months postoperatively. In spite of the efficacy of multimodal postoperative pain protocols, younger individuals with preoperative history of narcotic utilization needed additional opioids and were at a higher risk for adverse events and a greater LOS [1].

In 2019, Wilson et al. stated that multiple studies had shown that individuals taking opioids in the preoperative period were at elevated risk for adverse events following pTHA and pTKA [2]. However, the incidence and impact of opioid use disorder (OUD) among these individuals—both clinically and fiscally—were unknown. They investigated this relationship. The Nationwide Readmission Database (NRD) was utilized to identify individuals experiencing pTHA and pTKA

E. C. Rodríguez-Merchán (✉)
Department of Orthopedic Surgery, La Paz University Hospital, Madrid, Spain

from 2011 to 2015. The incidence of OUD in arthroplasty individuals increased 80% over the study period. OUD individuals had higher odds of periprosthetic joint infection (PJI), wound complication, prosthetic complication, and revision surgery. OUD patients also had longer LOSs (pTKA: +0.67 days; pTHA: +1.09 days), greater readmission, and increased 90-day costs (pTKA: +USD 3602; pTHA: USD + 4527). OUD represented a substantial risk factor for postoperative adverse event. It additionally conferred increased perioperative costs [2].

The purpose of this chapter is to analyze the impact of preoperative opioid use on revision TKA (rTKA) results.

4.2 Impact of Preoperative Long-Run Opioid Therapy on Patient Outcomes After pTKA

According to Kim et al., unsafe opioid distribution is a major concern among the pTKA population [3]. Perioperative opioid utilization had been demonstrated to be related to poorer results in individuals experiencing pTKA including longer LOS and discharges to extended care facilities. In a study with level 2 of evidence, they investigated the effects of preoperative chronic opioid utilization on perioperative quality results in pTKA individuals. A retrospective analysis was carried out on 338 consecutive pTKAs conducted at their hospital. Two groups were compared in this study—preoperative chronic opioid users and nonchronic opioid users. Fifty-four (16.0%) preoperative chronic opioid users were identified out of the total 338 individuals included in the study. Preoperative chronic opioid users experienced substantially longer LOS (2.9 versus 2.6 days). Individuals who remained persistent chronic users throughout the preoperative and postoperative stages showed a significantly longer LOS (3.4 days versus 2.5 days) compared with those who were no longer chronically using opioids by the 6 months postoperative period. By the 6 months postoperative time point, preoperative chronic users were consuming eight times the morphine equivalents (mg/day) compared with non-chronic users. Preoperative chronic opioid utilization was related to substantially higher usage patterns throughout the postoperative stages. Such opioid utilization patterns were related to longer LOS. Given that perioperative chronic opioid use has shown to negatively impact pTKA outcomes, future studies refining current perioperative management strategies are warranted [3].

In 2021, Wilson et al. affirmed that opioid utilization before pTKA was known to have detrimental influence on postoperative results [4]. However, whether or not the same was true for tramadol was unclear. In their study (level 3 of evidence), they tried to clarify the relationship between preoperative tramadol and postoperative adverse events. Individuals experiencing pTKA were identified and divided into cohorts based on preoperative medication status (i.e., opioid naïve, tramadol-only, or non-tramadol opioids). Patient demographics, comorbidities, and 90-day results were compared between cohorts. Revision rates were analyzed at 1 and 3 years postoperatively. 336,316 individuals were included and 23,097 (6.9%) were preoperative tramadol-only users. Tramadol-only individuals (versus opioid naïve) had increased odds of 90-day readmission, wound complication, and 3-year revision rates. However, when compared to the preoperative opioid cohorts, tramadol-only individuals had reduced odds of nearly all results. Over the study period, the number of individuals receiving preoperative opioids diminished, while the proportion of individuals prescribed tramadol-only augmented. While tramadol-only utilization had lower risk than traditional opioids, tramadol-only use preceding pTKA was associated with augmented percentages of readmission, wound adverse event, and revision surgery [4].

In 2021, Goplen et al. reported that up to 40% of individuals were receiving opioids at the time of pTKA in the United States despite evidence suggesting opioids were ineffective for pain associated with osteoarthritis and had significant risks [5]. They analyzed whether preoperative opioid users had worse knee pain and physical function results 1 year after pTKA than individuals who were opioid-naïve preoperatively; their secondary goal was to determine the prevalence of opioid utilization before and after pTKA. In a retrospective analysis of population-based data, Goplen et al. identified adult individuals who experienced pTKA between 2013 and 2015. They utilized multivariable linear regression to examine the association between preoperative opioid utilization and Western Ontario and McMaster Universities Osteoarthritis Index (WOMAC) pain and physical function scores 1 year after pTKA, adjusting for potentially confounding variables. Of the 1907 individuals, 592 (31%) had at least 1 opioid dispensed prior to pTKA, and 124 (6.5%) were classified as long-run opioid users. Long-run opioid users had worse adjusted WOMAC pain and physical function scores 1 year after pTKA than individuals who were opioid naive preoperatively. The majority (89 ([71.8%]) of individuals who were long-run opioid users preoperatively were dispensed opioids 180–360 days after pTKA, compared to 158 (12%) individuals who were opioid naive preoperatively. A significant number of individuals were dispensed opioids before and after pTKA, and individuals who received opioids preoperatively had worse adjusted pain and functional outcome scores 1 year after pTKA than individuals who were opioid naïve preoperatively [5].

In 2022, Singh et al. stated that the previous literature suggested that 25–30% of individuals who experience pTKA were utilizing opioids prior to their surgery [6]. In a study with level 3 of evidence, they investigated the impact of preoperative opioid utilization on clinical results and patient-reported outcome measures (PROMs) after pTKA. They retrospectively reviewed 329 individuals who experienced pTKA from 2019 to 2020, answered the preoperative opioid survey, and had accessible PROMs. Individuals were stratified into two cohorts based on whether they were taking opioids preoperatively or not: 26 individuals with preoperative opioid utilization (8%) and 303 individuals without preoperative opioid utilization (92%) were identified. Preoperative opioid users had a substantially longer LOS (2.74 versus 2.10) and surgical time (124.65 versus 105.69) and were more likely to be African-American (38.5 versus 14.2%) compared to preoperative opioid-naïve individuals. Postoperative Forgotten Joint Score (FJS-12) did not statistically differ between the two cohorts. While preoperative Knee Injury and Osteoarthritis Outcome Score for Joint Replacement (KOOS, JR) scores were significantly lower for preoperative opioid users (41.10 versus 46.63), they did not significantly differ postoperatively. Preoperative Veterans RAND-12 physical components (VR-12 PCS) did not statistically differ between the cohorts; however, both 3-month (33.87 versus 38.41) and 1-year (36.01 versus 44.73) scores were significantly lower for preoperative opioid users. Preoperative Veterans RAND-12 mental components (VR-12 MCS) was significantly lower for preoperative opioid users (46.06 versus 51.06), though not statistically different postoperatively. Preoperative opioid users had longer operative times and LOS compared to preoperatively opioid-naïve individuals. While both cohorts accomplished similar clinical benefits after pTKA, preoperative opioid users reported lower postoperative scores with respect to VR-12 PCS scores [6].

In 2022, Qin et al. compared perioperative events after pTKA among various degrees of preoperative opioid use [7]. In total, 84,569 individuals experiencing pTKA were identified and stratified by their preoperative opioid use based on number of prescriptions filled within 6 months of surgery (naïve 0 [50,561]; sporadic 1 [12,411]; chronic 2 or greater [21,687]). Adverse events rates (9.8% versus 8.9% versus 12.6%), need for supplemental oxygen (3% versus 3.1% versus 5.3%), mean LOS (2.1 versus 2.8 versus 3.5), and 90-day readmission (9.7% versus 10.8% versus 16.4%) substantially differed among cohorts. Only the chronic opioid use cohort was associated with substantially increased likelihood of adverse events, need for supplemental oxygen, and readmission [7].

In 2022, Huang et al. analyzed the prevalence of opioid use in a pTHA or pTKA cohort and its association with results [8]. About 837 pTHA or pTKA individuals prospectively completed Oxford scores, and Knee and Hip Osteoarthritis Outcome Score (KOOS/HOOS), and opioid utilization in the previous week before arthroplasty. Individuals repeated the baseline survey at 6 months, with additional questions regarding satisfaction. Opioid utilization was reported by 19% preoperatively and 7% at 6 months. Opioid utilization was 46% at 6 weeks and 10% at 6 months after pTKA and 16% at 6 weeks and 4% at 6 months after pTHA. Preoperative opioid utilization was associated with back pain, anxiety or depression and Oxford knee scores <30 in pTKA individuals, and females in pTHA individuals. There was no difference between preoperative opioid users and nonusers for satisfaction or KOOS or HOOS scores at 6 months. 77% of individuals taking opioids before surgery had ceased by 6 months, and 3% of preoperative nonusers reported opioid utilization at 6 months. Opioid use at 6 months was associated with preoperative use and lower 6-month Oxford scores. One in five utilized opioids prior to arthroplasty. Preoperative opioid use was the strongest risk factor for opioid use at 6 months, increasing odds 7–15 times. Prolonged opioid utilization was rarely found in the opioid naïve (<5% pTKA and 1% pTHA). Preoperative opioid utilization was not associated with inferior results or satisfaction [8].

In 2022, Smith et al. affirmed that chronic opioid utilization before pTKA has been implicated in adverse results [9]. They assessed clinical outcome measures and patient satisfaction in individuals with a history of preoperative chronic opioid utilization experiencing pTKA. A retrospective cohort study was carried out on 296 consecutive individuals experiencing pTKA. Seventy-four (25%) individuals were identified with chronic preoperative opioid utilization (study cohort; 22 males, 52 females). A 3:1 matched cohort ratio of control versus study cohort was used resulting in a control cohort consisting of 222 individuals (97 males, 125 females) without chronic opioid utilization before surgery. There was no statistically significant difference in age, body mass index (BMI), or follow-up. Average follow-up was 23.4 months in the control cohort and 23.6 months in the study cohort. Patient satisfaction at the most recent visit was 92.8% in the control cohort versus 83.8% in the chronic opioid cohort. Differences in PROMs comparing the control and study cohorts included Knee Society (KS) Function Score of 83.23 versus 75.31. The FJS of 63.7 versus 58 and the KS Knee Score of 89.5 versus 88.1 were not significant. Postoperative opioid usage for the control versus the study cohort was 62/222 (27.9%) versus 56/74 (75.7%) at 4–8 weeks and 4/222 (1.80%) versus 27/74 (36.5%) at 12 months. Overall adverse event occurrence was 18.9% in the study cohort versus 11.3% in the control cohort. Individuals with history of chronic preoperative opioid utilization had significantly lower patient satisfaction and KS Function scores and increased postoperative opioid usage at 1 year compared with individuals without a history of opioid utilization before pTKA [9].

4.3 Preoperative Opioid Utilization Is Associated with Early Revision Following TKA

In a study with level 3 of evidence published in 2017 by Ben-Ari et al., they stated that opioid utilization was endemic in the United States and was associated with morbidity and mortality [10]. However, the impact of long-run opioid utilization on joint replacement results remained unknown. They tested the hypothesis that utilization of opioids was associated with adverse results following pTKA. They carried out a retrospective analysis of individuals who had undergone pTKA within the US Veterans Affairs (VA) system over a 6-year period and had been followed for 1 year postoperatively. The length of time for which an opioid had been prescribed and the morphine equivalent dose were calculated for each individual. Individuals for whom opioids had been prescribed for >3 months in the year before the pTKA were assigned to the long-run opioid cohort. Of 32,636 individuals (94.4% male; mean age 64.45 years) who experienced pTKA, 12,772 (39.1%) were in the long-run opioid cohort, and 734 (2.2%) had a revision within a year following the pTKA. Chronic kidney disease, diabetes, and long-run opioid utilization were associated with revision within 1 year and were also the leading factors associated with a revision at any time following the index TKA. There was no relationship between long-run utilization of opioids and the specific cause for knee revision. Long-run opioid utilization before pTKA was associated with an increased risk of knee revision during the first year after pTKA among predominantly male individuals treated in the VA system [10].

According to Bedard et al. (2018), few studies had assessed the impact of preoperative opioid utilization on risk of subsequent revision following pTKA [11]. Therefore, they studied whether preoperative opioid utilization was associated with an increased risk of early rTKA. The Humana administrative claims database was queried to identify individuals who experienced unilateral pTKA during the years 2007–2015. Individuals were tracked for the occurrence of an ipsilateral revision procedure within 2 years. Preoperative opioid utilization was defined as having an opioid prescription filled within the 3 months prior to TKA. Age, sex, diabetes, obesity, chronic kidney disease, and anxiety/depression were also analyzed. A total of 35,894 pTKA individuals were identified and 1.2% ($N = 413$) had a rTKA procedure within 2 years. 29.2% of individuals filled an opioid prescription within the 3 months prior to TKA. Preoperative opioid users were substantially more likely to experience early rTKA (1.6% versus 1%). Preoperative opioid utilization, younger age, obesity, and smoking were associated with early rTKA. This study identified preoperative opioid utilization as being independently associated with a greater risk for an early rTKA. Younger age, obesity, and smoking were also associated with elevated risk. These findings supported efforts to diminish inappropriate opioid prescribing [11].

4.4 Preoperative Opioid Utilization Is Associated with Higher Readmission and Revision Rates in TKA

In a study with level 4 of evidence published in 2018 by Weick et al., they affirmed that prescription opioid utilization was epidemic in the United States. In fact, an association had been shown between preoperative opioid utilization and increased healthcare use following abdominal surgeries. Given that pTKA and pTHA were two of the most common surgical procedures in the United States, Weick et al. analyzed the association of preoperative opioid utilization with 30-day readmission and early revision rates [12]. They reviewed 2003 to 2014 data from two Truven Health MarketScan databases (commercial insurance and Medicare plus commercial supplemental insurance). Individuals were included if they had a Current Procedural Terminology (CPT) code for pTKA or pTHA and were continuously enrolled in the database for at least 6 months before the index procedure. Preoperative opioid prescriptions were identified utilizing National Drug Codes (NDCs). Rates of 30-day readmissions and revision arthroplasty were identified and compared among individuals with stratified durations of preoperative opioid utilization in the 6 months preceding pTKA or pTHA. The study included 324,154 individuals in the 1-year follow-up cohort and 159,822 individuals in the 3-year follow-up cohort. Opioid-naive pTKA individuals had a lower revision rate than did those with >60 days of preoperative opioid utilization (1-year group, 1.07% compared with 2.14%; 3-year group, 2.58% compared with 5% (Figs. 4.1 and 4.2). A similar trend was observed among pTHA individuals (1 year, 0.38% compared with 1.10%; 3 year, 1.24% compared with 2.99%). These trends persisted after adjusting for age, sex, and Charlson Comorbidity Index (CCI). The 30-day readmission rate after pTKA or pTHA was substantially lower for individuals with no preoperative opioid utilization compared with those with >60 days of preoperative opioid utilization (pTKA, 4.82%

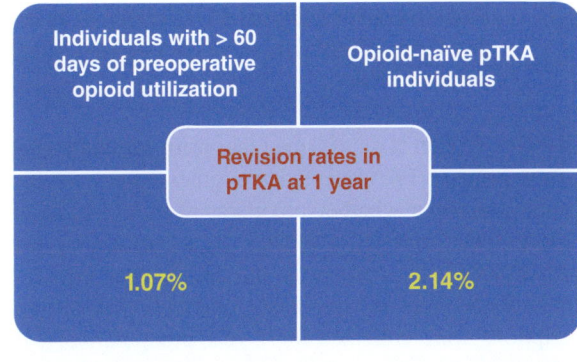

Fig. 4.1 Revision rates at 1 year. Comparison between opioid-naïve primary total knee arthroplasty (pTKA) patients and patients with >60 days of preoperative opioid use [12]

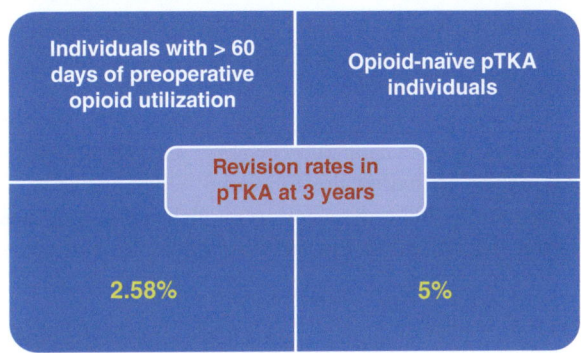

Fig. 4.2 Revision rates at 3 years. Comparison between opioid-naïve primary total knee arthroplasty (pTKA) patients and patients with >60 days of preoperative opioid use [12]

compared with 6.17%; pTHA, 3.71% compared with 5.85%). Again, this association persisted after adjusting for age, sex, and CCI. Preoperative opioid utilization was associated with substantially augmented risk of early revision and substantially augmented risk of 30-day readmission following TKA and THA. This study showed the augmented risk of poor results and augmented postoperative healthcare use for individuals with long-run opioid utilization before pTHA and pTKA [12].

4.5 A Risk Calculator Utilizing Preoperative Opioids for Prediction of rTKA

In 2018, Starr et al. stated that no risk calculator including opioid utilization or other risk factors was currently accessible for predicting rTKA [13]. They retrospectively analyzed medical records of Veterans Affairs individuals who experienced TKA from January 1, 2006, to January 1, 2012. Individuals were followed until January 1, 2013. Chronic opioid utilization was defined as opioid use for ≥3 months preoperatively. Totally, 32,297 individuals were included. A risk calculator was generated with a mean absolute error of 0.1% at 1 year and 3.6% at 5 years. Chronic opioid utilization was a significant predictor of rTKA [13].

4.6 Preoperative Opioid Utilization Is a Risk Factor for Complication and Increased Healthcare Use After rTKA

In 2020, Wilson et al. affirmed that prior literature suggested that opioid utilization before primary TKA resulted in augmented risk for complication [14]. Despite this, it was unknown whether preoperative opioid utilization increased risk following rTKA. That was why Wilson et al. examined this relationship. The Truven MarketScan® database was utilized to perform a retrospective cohort study. Individuals experiencing rTKA for aseptic indication were identified. Opioid prescriptions were collected for 1 year preoperatively. Individuals were divided into cohorts based on the number of prescriptions received preoperatively. Individuals who had an "opioid holiday" (6 months of opioid-naïve period after prior use) were also analyzed. In the year preceding surgery, 84% of individuals received an opioid prescription. Compared to opioid-naïve individuals, continuous preoperative utilization was associated with higher odds of PJI, venous thromboembolism, opioid overdose, and revision surgery (Fig. 4.3). Similarly, healthcare use was higher in this cohort including the following: extended LOS, nonhome discharge, 90-day readmission, and emergency room visits (Fig. 4.4). The opioid holiday seemed to confer risk reduction. Preoperative opioid utilization preceding rTKA was common

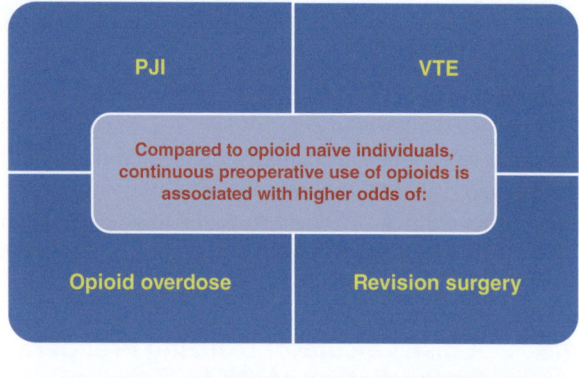

Fig. 4.3 Continuous preoperative use of opioids is associated with higher odds of adverse events after revision total knee arthroplasty (rTKA) [14]. *PJI* Periprosthetic joint infection, *VTE* Venous thromboembolism

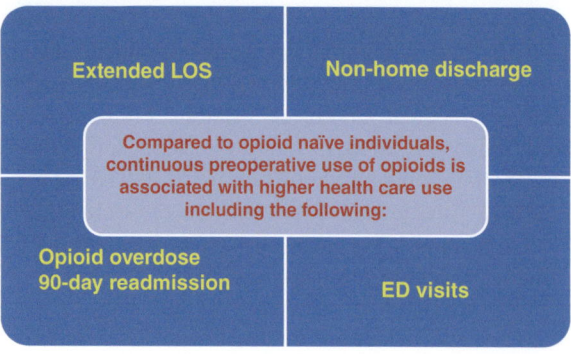

Fig. 4.4 Continuous preoperative use of opioids is associated with higher healthcare use after revision total knee arthroplasty (rTKA) [14]. *LOS* Length of stay, *ED* Emergency department

and was associated with adverse events following surgery. An opioid holiday seemed to provide risk reduction and suggested that opioid utilization might be a modifiable risk factor [14].

4.7 Impact of Preoperative Opioid Utilization on PROMs After rTKA

In 2023, Ingall et al. stated that prior studies have characterized the deleterious effects of narcotic utilization in individuals experiencing pTKA [15]. However, information on the effect of narcotic utilization in the revision surgery setting remained limited. They analyzed the effect of active narcotic utilization at the time of rTKA on PROMs. Three-hundred and thirty consecutive individuals who experienced rTKA and completed both pre- and postoperative PROMs were identified. Pre- and postoperative Knee Injury and Osteoarthritis Outcome Score-Physical Function (KOOS-PS), patient-reported outcomes measurement information system short form (PROMIS SF) physical, PROMIS SF mental, and physical SF 10A scores were assessed. Opioid utilization was identified by the medication reconciliation on the day of surgery. Propensity score-matched opioid users had substantially lower preoperative PROMs than the nonuser for KOOS-PS (45.2 versus 53.8), PROMIS SF physical (37.2 versus 42.5), PROMIS SF mental (44.2 versus 51.3), and physical SF 10A (34.1 versus 36.8). Postoperatively, opioid users showed substantially lower scores across all PROMs: KOOS-PS (59.2 versus 67.2), PROMIS SF physical (43.2 versus 52.4), PROMIS SF mental (47.5 versus 58.9), and physical SF 10A (40.5 versus 49.4). Propensity score-matched opioid users showed a substantially smaller absolute increase in scores for PROMIS SF Physical and Physical SF 10A, as well as an augmented hospital LOS. Individuals who were actively taking opioids at the time of rTKA reported substantially lower preoperative and postoperative outcome scores. These individuals were more likely to have longer LOSs. The apparent negative impact on PROMs following rTKA provided clinically useful data for surgeons in engaging individuals in a preoperative counseling regarding narcotic utilization before rTKA to optimize results [15].

4.8 Conclusions

Long-run opioid utilization before pTKA is associated with an increased risk of knee revision during the first year after pTKA among predominantly male individuals. Preoperative opioid utilization is independently associated with a greater risk for an early rTKA. A study has shown that preoperative opioid utilization is associated with substantially augmented risk of early revision and substantially augmented risk of 30-day readmission following TKA. The aforementioned study showed the augmented risk of poor results and augmented postoperative healthcare use for individuals with long-run opioid utilization before pTKA. In another report, chronic opioid utilization (defined as opioid use for ≥ 3 months preoperatively) was a significant predictor of rTKA. Other authors found that continuous preoperative utilization before rTKA was associated with higher odds of adverse events. This included PJI, VTE, opioid overdose, and revision surgery. Besides, healthcare use was higher in this cohort including the following: extended LOS, nonhome discharge, 90-day readmission, and emergency room visits. The opioid holiday (6 months of opioid-naïve period after prior use) seemed to confer risk reduction. Finally, other authors encountered that individuals who were actively taking opioids at the time of rTKA reported substantially lower preoperative and postoperative outcome scores. These individuals were more likely to have longer LOSs.

References

1. Rozell JC, Courtney PM, Dattilo JR, Wu CH, Lee GC. Preoperative opiate use independently predicts narcotic consumption and complications after total joint arthroplasty. J Arthroplast. 2017;32(9):2658–62. https://doi.org/10.1016/j.arth.2017.04.002.
2. Wilson JM, Farley KX, Aizpuru M, Wagner ER, Bradbury TL, Guild GN. The impact of preoperative opioid use disorder on complications and costs following primary total hip and knee arthroplasty. Adv Orthop. 2019;2019:9319480. https://doi.org/10.1155/2019/9319480.
3. Kim K, Chen K, Anoushiravani AA, Roof M, Long WJ, Schwarzkopf R. Preoperative chronic opioid use and its effects on total knee arthroplasty outcomes. J Knee Surg. 2020;33(3):306–13. https://doi.org/10.1055/s-0039-1678538.
4. Wilson JM, Schwartz AM, Farley KX, Erens GA, Bradbury TL, Guild GN. The impact of preoperative tramadol-only use on outcomes following total knee arthroplasty—is tramadol different than traditional opioids? Knee. 2021;28:131–8. https://doi.org/10.1016/j.knee.2020.11.003.
5. Goplen CM, Kang SH, Randell JR, Jones CA, Voaklander DC, Churchill TA, et al. Effect of preoperative long-term opioid therapy on patient outcomes after total knee arthroplasty: an analysis of multicentre population-based administrative data. Can J Surg. 2021;64(2):E135–43. https://doi.org/10.1503/cjs.007319.
6. Singh V, Fiedler B, Sicat CS, Bi AS, Slover JD, Long WJ, et al. Impact of preoperative opioid use on patient-reported outcomes following primary total knee arthroplasty. Eur J Orthop Surg Traumatol. 2023;33(4):1283–90. https://doi.org/10.1007/s00590-022-03297-w.
7. Qin CD, Vatti L, Qin MM, Lee CS, Athiviraham A. The relationship between preoperative opioid use and adverse events following total knee arthroplasty. J Surg Orthop Adv. 2022;31(2):100–3.
8. Huang P, Brownrigg J, Roe J, Carmody D, Pinczewski L, Gooden B, et al. Opioid use and patient outcomes in an Australian hip and knee arthroplasty cohort. ANZ J Surg. 2022;92(9):2261–8. https://doi.org/10.1111/ans.17969.
9. Smith AF, Smith NS, Smith LS, Yakkanti MR, Malkani AL. Does preoperative opioid consumption influence patient satisfaction following total knee arthroplasty? J Knee Surg. 2023;36(13):1374–9. https://doi.org/10.1055/a-1946-6217.
10. Ben-Ari A, Chansky H, Rozet I. Preoperative opioid use is associated with early revision after total knee arthroplasty: a study of male patients treated in the veterans affairs system. J Bone Joint Surg Am. 2017;99(1):1–9. https://doi.org/10.2106/JBJS.16.00167.
11. Bedard NA, DeMik DE, Dowdle SB, Owens JM, Liu SS, Callaghan JJ. Preoperative opioid use and its association with early revision of total knee arthroplasty. J Arthroplast. 2018;33(11):3520–3. https://doi.org/10.1016/j.arth.2018.06.005.
12. Weick J, Bawa H, Dirschl DR, Luu HH. Preoperative opioid use is associated with higher readmission and revision rates in total knee and total hip arthroplasty. J Bone Joint Surg Am. 2018;100(14):1171–6. https://doi.org/10.2106/JBJS.17.01414.

13. Starr J, Rozet I, Ben-Ari A. A risk calculator using preoperative opioids for prediction of total knee revision arthroplasty. Clin J Pain. 2018;34(4):328–31. https://doi.org/10.1097/AJP.0000000000000544.
14. Wilson JM, Farley KX, Bradbury TL, Erens GA, Guild GN. Preoperative opioid use is a risk factor for complication and increased healthcare utilization following revision total knee arthroplasty. Knee. 2020;27(4):1121–7. https://doi.org/10.1016/j.knee.2020.05.013.
15. Ingall E, Klemt C, Melnic CM, Cohen-Levy WB, Tirumala V, Kwon YM. Impact of preoperative opioid use on patient-reported outcomes after revision total knee arthroplasty: a propensity matched analysis. J Knee Surg. 2023;36(2):115–20. https://doi.org/10.1055/s-0041-1729966.

Patient Satisfaction After Revision Total Knee Arthroplasty

5

E. Carlos Rodríguez-Merchán

5.1 Introduction

The published dissatisfaction percentage following primary total knee arthroplasty (pTKA) ranges between 15% and 25% [1]. In a study with level 4 of evidence published in 2023, Gousopoulos et al. found that at a minimum follow-up of 2 years after custom pTKA combined with "personalized alignment," 94% of individuals were either satisfied or very satisfied and the PASS (patient acceptable symptom state) criteria were accomplished in 89% for OKS (Oxford Knee Score) and 85% for FJS (Forgotten Joint Score), all of which compared favorably to reported result of off-the-shelf pTKA [2].

In 2023, Oledeji et al. presented surgical techniques utilized in conversion total knee arthroplasty (TKA) after early failure of large osteochondral allograft joint replacement and compared postoperative patient reported outcomes measures (PROMs) and satisfaction scores with a contemporary pTKA group. It was found that conversion TKA after failed biological replacement was associated with similar postoperative improvement as in pTKA. Lower patient reported conversion TKA satisfaction was associated with lower postoperative KOOS-JR (Knee Injury and Osteoarthritis Outcome Score for Joint Replacement) scores [3].

The purpose of this chapter is to analyze patient satisfaction after revision total knee arthroplasty (rTKA).

E. C. Rodríguez-Merchán (✉)
Department of Orthopedic Surgery, La Paz University Hospital, Madrid, Spain

© The Author(s), under exclusive license to Springer Nature Switzerland AG 2024
E. C. Rodríguez-Merchán (ed.), *Advances in Revision Total Knee Arthroplasty*, https://doi.org/10.1007/978-3-031-60445-4_5

5.2 Evaluation of Patient Satisfaction Following Revision TKA

According to Quinn et al., patient satisfaction following revision TKA (rTKA) is poorly described within the literature [4]. They investigated postoperative satisfaction of rTKA individuals utilizing a single prosthesis, at a single institution. Patient satisfaction was evaluated utilizing structured telephone assessment questionnaires and review of orthopedic/hospital records. The impact of patient and surgical characteristics on satisfaction was evaluated utilizing correlation coefficients and binary logistic regression in SPSS. Two hundred and two rTKAs were carried out in 178 individuals between 2004 and 2015 inclusive. One hundred and twenty-four individuals (143 rTKAs) were contactable to complete satisfaction evaluation. Figure 5.1 summarizes the rates of patient satisfaction after rTKA [4]. The Mahomed satisfaction scale (Table 5.1) [5] results showed a mean score of 87.7. High positive correlation was encountered between evaluation tools. Factors contributing to satisfaction are shown in Fig. 5.2 [4]. This group showed high patient satisfaction rate following rTKA, using simple and dependable outcome measurement tools. Quinn et al. observed a high positive correlation between methods of evaluation and

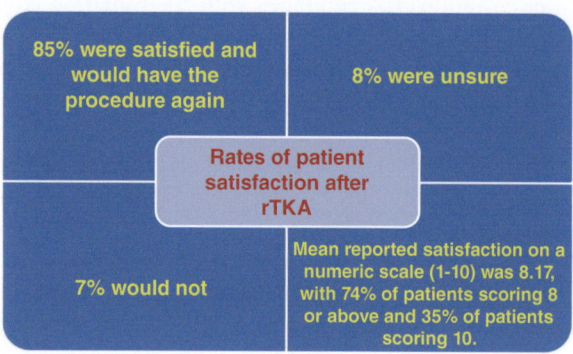

Fig. 5.1 Rates of satisfaction after revision total knee arthroplasty (rTKA)

Table 5.1 The Mahomed satisfaction scale [5]

Items	Very satisfied	Somewhat satisfied	Somewhat dissatisfied	Very dissatisfied
Patients' overall satisfaction with surgery	100 points	75 points	50 points	25 points
The extent of pain relief	100 points	75 points	50 points	25 points
The ability to perform home or yard work	100 points	75 points	50 points	25 points
The ability to perform recreational activities	100 points	75 points	50 points	25 points

Items are scored on a 4-point Likert scale with response categories consisting of very satisfied (100 points), somewhat satisfied (75 points), somewhat dissatisfied (50 points), and very dissatisfied (25 points). The scale score is the unweighted mean of the scores from the individual items, ranging from 25 to 100 per item (with 100 being most satisfied)

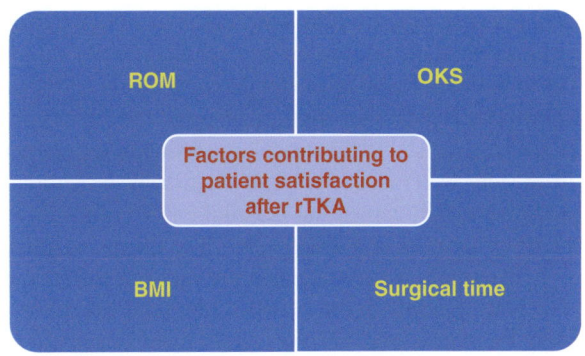

Fig. 5.2 Factors contributing to satisfaction after revision total knee arthroplasty (rTKA). *ROM* Range of motion, *OKS* Oxford Knee Score, *BMI* Body mass index

moderate positive correlation between satisfaction and functional results. These findings contributed to the understanding of satisfaction in rTKA individuals, which might assist in informing individuals of expected postoperative results [4].

5.3 PROMs and Satisfaction 1–3 Years After rTKA for Unexplained Pain Versus Aseptic Loosening

In a cross-sectional case-control study published in 2023, Ardnt et al. compared PROMs and satisfaction 1 to 3 years after rTKAs for the indications of unexplained pain versus aseptic loosening [6]. They included 384 individuals experiencing rTKA for the indications of unexplained pain and aseptic loosening from January 1, 2018, to December 31, 2020, from the Danish Knee Arthroplasty Register. A total of 81 individuals were revised for unexplained pain and 303 for aseptic loosening. Questionnaires including PROMs [OKS, EuroQol (EQ-5D-5L), and FJS] and satisfaction with the surgery on a 0–100 scale (100 = not satisfied; 0 = very satisfied) were sent to digitally secured mailboxes. Time from revision to data collection was a median 3.1 years (range, 1.4–4.4 years). Median OKS was 25 versus 31, 1–3 years after revisions for unexplained pain versus aseptic loosening. Median EQ-5D-5L was 0.6 versus 0.8 for unexplained pain versus aseptic loosening. Median FJS was 50 versus 50 for unexplained pain versus aseptic loosening. Satisfaction was 75 for unexplained pain and 50 for aseptic loosening. Individuals experiencing rTKA for the indication of unexplained pain had worse outcomes on PROMs than those revised for aseptic loosening. Likewise, individuals revised for unexplained pain were less satisfied compared to individuals revised for aseptic loosening [6].

5.4 Patient's Satisfaction Following rTKA Using a Modified Hybrid Cementing Technique

In a study with level 3 of evidence published in 2020, Kim et al. stated that there had been no studies comparing PROMs including end-of-stem tip pain and patient satisfaction based on the use of cementing techniques in rTKA [7]. Kim et al. compared end-of-stem tip pain and PROMs with hybrid and modified hybrid cementing techniques in rTKAs. Sixty-two cases of rTKA performed were divided into two cohorts based on the cementing technique with a minimum follow-up of 2 years. Two types of cementing technique for femoral and tibial stems were utilized as follows: (1) a hybrid cementing technique (33 cases), in which cement was applied immediately distal to the modular junction of the stem and the component while the distal stem was press-fitted into the diaphysis without utilizing cement, and (2) a modified hybrid cementing technique (29 cases), in which cement was applied to the tip of femoral and tibial stems. The thigh and shin were evaluated for the end-of-stem tip pain. Patient satisfaction was assessed based on the satisfaction items of New Knee Society Score (nKSS). Modified hybrid cementing substantially diminished the percentage of individuals manifesting shin pain (3.4% versus 24.2%). Individuals managed with the modified hybrid cementing technique exhibited a higher satisfaction percentage. Multivariate logistic regression analysis demonstrated an increase in the odds of satisfaction 32.686-fold in individuals without pain at the end-of-stem tip in the shin and 9.261-fold in individuals managed with the modified hybrid cementing technique. The modified hybrid cementing technique for fixation of long-stem in rTKAs diminished the end-of-stem tip pain in the shin, leading to substantially greater satisfaction compared with the hybrid cementing technique following rTKA [7].

5.5 Satisfaction Rates Are Low Following rTKA in Asians Despite Improvements in PROMs

In 2020, Abd Razak et al. assessed results and satisfaction percentages after rTKA in an Asian population [8]. Registry information of individuals who experienced rTKA from 2006 to 2010 and had completed 5 years of follow-up was analyzed. Flexion range, OKS, KSS, the Short-Form 36 (SF-36), and satisfaction percentages were evaluated for improvement from preoperative values, as well as by the minimum clinically important difference (MCID) criterion. rTKA was carried out in 163 individuals. There were substantial improvements found at 2 years postoperatively, and these were sustained up to 5 years. The MCID criterion for KSS, OKS, and SF-36 physical component score was met at 2 and 5 years postoperatively. The rate of adverse events was 3.7% at a mean follow-up of 8.4 years. A total of 121 individuals (74.2%) were satisfied at 5 years postoperatively. rTKA led to significantly improved PROMs with a low complication rate of 3.7% at a minimum of 5-year follow-up [8].

5.6 rTKA Is Associated with Lower Hospital Consumer Assessment of Healthcare Providers and Systems Patient Satisfaction Scores Compared with pTKA

In a study with level 3 of evidence published in 2022, Mercier et al. compared the survey results of Hospital Consumer Assessment of Healthcare Providers and Systems (HCAHPS) between individuals who experienced pTKA versus rTKA. rTKA individuals showed lower total top-box rates (76.13% versus 79.22%)

and lower scores on the care from doctors' subsection (66.28% versus 83.65%) of the HCAHPS survey. rTKA was associated with lower total HCAHPS scores and rated care from doctors. This suggested that HCAHPS scores might be biased by factors outside the surgeon's control, such as the complexity associated with rTKA [9].

5.7 Conclusions

It has been published that after rTKA 85% of individuals were satisfied and would have the procedure again, 8% were unsure, and 7% would not. The mean reported satisfaction on a numerical scale (1–10) was 8.17 (range 1–10), with 74% of individuals scoring 8 or above, and 35% of individuals scoring 10. In a study, individuals experiencing rTKA for the indication of unexplained pain had worse results on PROMs than those revised for aseptic loosening. Other authors encountered that at 5 years postoperatively 74.2% of individuals were satisfied and that rTKA led to significantly improved PROMs with a low complication rate of 3.7%.

References

1. Rodriguez-Merchan EC. Patient satisfaction following primary total knee arthroplasty: contributing factors. Arch Bone Jt Surg. 2021;9(4):379–86. https://doi.org/10.22038/abjs.2020.46395.2274.
2. Gousopoulos L, Dobbelaere A, Ratano S, Bondoux L, Tibesku CO, Aït-Si-Selmi T, et al. Custom total knee arthroplasty combined with personalised alignment grants 94% patient satisfaction at minimum follow-up of 2 years. Knee Surg Sports Traumatol Arthrosc. 2023;31(4):1276–83. https://doi.org/10.1007/s00167-023-07318-x.
3. Oladeji LO, Albracht BG, Keeney JA. Conversion total knee arthroplasty after failed osteochondral allograft reconstruction: similar functional performance with lower patient satisfaction. J Arthroplast. 2023;38(6):1045–51. https://doi.org/10.1016/j.arth.2023.02.084.
4. Quinn J, Jones P, Randle R. Assessment of patient satisfaction following revision total knee arthroplasty. ANZ J Surg. 2023;93(4):995–1000. https://doi.org/10.1111/ans.18375.
5. Mahomed N, Gandhi R, Daltroy L, Katz JN. The self-administered patient satisfaction scale for primary hip and knee arthroplasty. Arthritis. 2011;2011:591253. https://doi.org/10.1155/2011/591253.
6. Arndt KB, Schrøder HM, Troelsen A, Lindberg-Larsen M. Patient-reported outcomes and satisfaction 1 to 3 years after revisions of total knee arthroplasties for unexplained pain versus aseptic loosening. J Arthroplast. 2023;38(3):535–540.e3. https://doi.org/10.1016/j.arth.2022.10.019.
7. Kim MS, Koh IJ, Sohn S, Park HC, In Y. Modified hybrid cementing technique reduces stem tip pain and improves patient's satisfaction after revision total knee arthroplasty. J Orthop Surg Res. 2020;15(1):393. https://doi.org/10.1186/s13018-020-01921-1.
8. Bin Abd Razak HR, Lee JHM, Tan SM, Chong HC, Lo NN, Yeo SJ. Satisfaction rates are low following revision total knee arthroplasty in Asians despite improvements in patient-reported outcome measures. J Knee Surg. 2020;33(10):1041–6. https://doi.org/10.1055/s-0039-1692629.
9. Mercier MR, Galivanche AR, Pathak N, Mets EJ, Molho DA, Elaydi AH, et al. Revision total hip and knee arthroplasty are associated with lower hospital consumer assessment of healthcare providers and systems patient satisfaction scores compared with primary arthroplasty. J Am Acad Orthop Surg. 2022;30(3):e336–46. https://doi.org/10.5435/JAAOS-D-21-00839.

Isolated Versus Full-Component Revision in Total Knee Arthroplasty for Aseptic Loosening

E. Carlos Rodríguez-Merchán

6.1 Introduction

According to Apinyankul et al., revision of both femoral and tibial components of a total knee arthroplasty (TKA) for aseptic loosening has favorable results. Revision of only one loose component with retention of others has shorter operative time and lower cost; however, implant survivorship and clinical results of these different surgical procedures are unclear [1]. The purpose of this chapter is to review the literature that compared isolated versus full-component revision in TKA for aseptic loosening.

6.2 Comparison Between Isolated Polyethylene Bearing Exchange Versus Full-Component Revision in TKA for Aseptic Loosening

In 2002, Babis et al. stated that in spite of improvements in the design and manufacturing of the components utilized in TKA, wear of the polyethylene (PE) bearing remained a potential source of failure. One theoretical advantage of modular tibial implants is that, when the components are well fixed, individuals with wear or instability of the PE bearing can be treated with isolated tibial polyethylene insert exchange (ITPIE) [2]. They evaluated the outcomes of ITPIE during revision surgery in a relatively large, consecutive group of individuals. From 1985 through 1997, they carried out 56 ITPIEs in 55 individuals (29 men [one man had bilateral revision] and 26 women; mean age, 66 years) primarily because of wear or instability. Individuals with loosening of any of the components, a history of infection,

E. C. Rodríguez-Merchán (✉)
Department of Orthopedic Surgery, La Paz University Hospital, Madrid, Spain

© The Author(s), under exclusive license to Springer Nature Switzerland AG 2024
E. C. Rodríguez-Merchán (ed.), *Advances in Revision Total Knee Arthroplasty*, https://doi.org/10.1007/978-3-031-60445-4_6

severe stiffness of the knee, recognized malposition of any component, or problems with the extensor mechanism were excluded. Twelve knees had undergone one, two, or three prior revisions. The duration of follow-up averaged 8.3 years (range, 1.6–16.2 years) after the index TKA and 4.6 years (range, 2–14 years) after the revision. The mean Knee Society knee and function scores improved from 56 and 50.9 points before the revision to 76 and 59 points at the time of final follow-up. Fourteen (25%) of the 56 knees subsequently needed re-revision at a mean of only 3 years (range, 0.5–6.8 years) after the ITPIE. The cumulative survival rate at 5.5 years was 63.5%. Of the 27 knees with preoperative instability, eight were re-revised, and another four were considered failures because of severe pain. Of the 24 knees that were treated with the index revision because of wear of the PE bearing, five were re-revised. Besides, one extremity in this group was amputated above the knee as a result of chronic osteomyelitis of the ankle concomitant with chronic pain at the site of the TKA, and another two PE bearings were considered failures because of severe pain. Babis et al. concluded that ITPIE resulted in a surprisingly high percentage of early failure. Therefore, the recommended that ITPIE should be undertaken with caution [2].

In a study with level 2 of evidence published in 2010, Wilson et al. affirmed that TKA utilizing a modular design allowed ITPIE as a treatment alternative for isolated PE failure [3]. They asked whether ITPIE in selected individuals would provide high survivorship and identified factors predicting success or failure. They retrospectively reviewed 42 individuals (42 knees) who experienced ITPIE for instability, stiffness, or aseptic effusions after TKA. All individuals had well-aligned and well-fixed components documented by radiographs and intraoperative assessment. Wilson et al. determined whether individuals had been revised and assessed unrevised individuals utilizing the Knee Society rating system. The minimum follow-up was 2 years (average, 5.6 years; range, 2–11 years). Twelve individuals (29%) experienced subsequent revision of their ITPIE (58% survivorship at 11 years). Average time to revision was 3 years. Although mean Knee Society Scores improved, nine of the 30 unrevised individuals (30%) had persistent pain at follow-up. Time from index TKA to ITPIE was associated with result; ITPIE less than 3 years from index TKA was 3.8 times more likely to experience re-revision than ITPIE more than 3 years from index TKA. The conclusion was that ITPIE for failed TKA was associated with unpredictable results. ITPIE, even with well-defined and narrow indications, should be performed with caution. The longer the initial components performed successfully prior to ITPIE, the greater the likelihood of success following ITPIE.

In 2018, Cooper et al. affirmed that symptomatic instability after TKA was an important cause of early failure. Most publications recommended component revision as the preferred treatment because of poor results and high failure rates with ITPIE. However, these ideas had not been tested in modern implant systems that allow insert constraint to be increased [4]. They retrospectively reviewed 90 individuals with minimum 2-year (mean 3.7 years) follow-up who experienced rTKA for instability. Mean age was 62 years (range, 41–83 years), and 73% of patients were women. Forty percent of individuals were treated with ITPIE when standardized preoperative and intraoperative criteria were met; 60% experienced revision of one or both components when these criteria were not met. Individuals experienced substantial improvements in Knee Society knee (48.4–82.6) and function (49–81) scores. There were no substantial differences in improvements in Knee Society Knee Scores (KSKS) (38.1 versus 33.1), Knee Society Function Scores (KSFS) (36 versus 34), or range of motion (ROM) (5° versus 6°) between those treated with ITPIE and component revision. Failure rates were 19.4% in the ITPIE cohort versus 18.5% in the component revision cohort. Re-revision rates were substantially lower (6.3% versus 30.8%) when PE insert constraint was increased. In selected individuals, ITPIE was not inferior to component revision at addressing symptomatic instability after TKA. Grade of constraint should be augmented whenever possible during revision surgery for instability.

In 2021, Tetreaut et al. analyzed the outcomes of ITPIE during rTKA [5]. From 1985 to 2016, 270 ITPIEs were carried out for instability (55%, $N = 148$), PE wear (39%, $N = 105$), insert fracture/dissociation (5%, $N = 14$), or stiffness (1%, $N = 3$). Individuals with component loosening, implant malposition, infection, and extensor mechanism problems were excluded. Survivorship free of any re-revision was 68% at 10 years. For the indication of insert wear, survivorship free of any re-revision at 10 years was 74%. Re-revisions were more frequent for index diagnoses other than wear, with 10-year survivorships of 69% for instability and 37% for insert fracture/dissociation. Following ITPIE for wear, the most frequent reason for re-revision was aseptic loosening (33%, $N = 7$). For other indications, the most frequent reason for re-revision was recurrence of the original diagnosis. Mean Knee Society Scores (KSS) improved from 54 (0–94) preoperatively to 77 (38–94) at 10 years. Following ITPIE, the risk and reasons for re-revision correlated with preoperative indications. The best outcomes were for PE wear. For other diagnoses, the re-revision percentage was higher, and the failure mode was most frequently recurrence of the original indication for the rTKA [5].

In 2022, Alexander et al. stated that ITPIE as a treatment for instability and PE wear after TKA remained controversial with studies reporting varied outcomes. They assessed the survival and results of ITPIE carried out for treatment of instability with or without PE wear after TKA [6]. They analyzed 364 individuals (390 knees) treated with ITPIE for instability and/or PE wear after TKA between 1997 and 2019. Mean age was 66.8 years, mean body mass index (BMI) was 33.8 kg/m^2, and 59% of individuals were female. ITPIE for infection, tibiofemoral aseptic loosening, arthrofibrosis, poor wound healing, and extensor mechanism failure were excluded. All individuals had well-fixed and well-aligned components before surgery. Mean follow-up was 5.9 years. Knee Society Clinical (KSC) scores improved preoperatively from 55 to 76 postoperatively. Thirty knees (7.7%) needed re-revision: 15 (3.8%) for ongoing instability, seven aseptic loosening, three infection, two patellofemoral mal-tracking, one patellar fracture, one metal allergy, and one revised elsewhere for cause unknown. Kaplan-Meier analysis revealed survival of 93.1% at 5 years, 84.7% at 10 years, and 80.5% at 21 years (Fig. 6.1). ITPIE was a

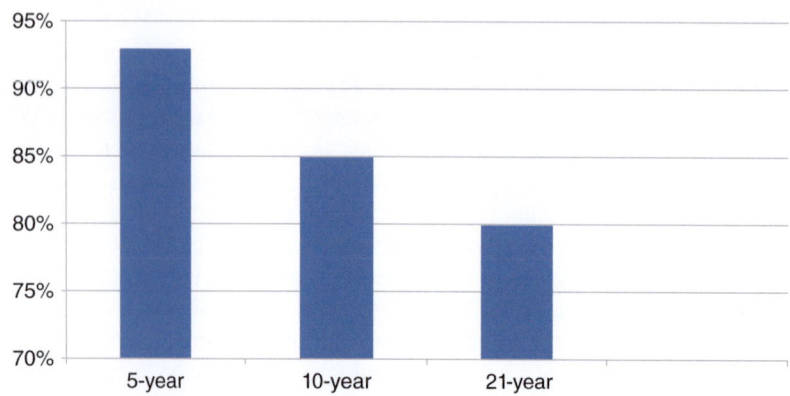

Fig. 6.1 Isolated tibial polyethylene insert exchange (ITPIE) carried out for treatment of instability with or without polyethylene (PE) wear after total knee arthroplasty (TKA): Kaplan-Meier analysis

dependable treatment for instability and/or PE wear following TKA in the presence of well-fixed and well-aligned components with good survival and clinical improvement. The less invasive nature and diminished risk for bone loss made it an attractive alternative versus full revision [6].

6.3 Comparison Between Clinical and Radiographic Outcomes of Partial-Component Versus Full-Component rTKA

In a study with level 3 of evidence published in 2004, Fehring et al. compared the clinical and radiographic outcomes of partial-component versus full-component rTKA [7]. A retrospective review was utilized to identify individuals who experienced partial rTKA. Only isolated femoral or tibial revisions were included. From 1986 to 2000, 448 rTKAs were done. Seventy-seven partial revisions were done. Three were excluded for a diagnosis of infection. The average follow-up was 63 months. The average KSS for full-component revisions was 85 compared with 79 for partial revisions. This difference was significant. The average KSS for those individuals who experienced a full revision for instability was 85 compared with 63 for partial revision. The average KSS for those individuals who experienced a full revision for wear-related problems was 88 compared with 78 for partial revisions. The efficacy of partial revision has not been established in rTKA. Care should be taken when considering partial revision for instability or wear-related problems [7].

In a study with level 3 of evidence published in 2021, Lee et al. stated that an isolated tibial component revision could be a treatment for isolated tibial side loosening; however, few studies had demonstrated its efficacy [8]. They compared the clinical and radiological results between isolated (tibial component) and total (femoral and tibial component) rTKA. Between January 2008 and February 2017, 31 individuals experienced rTKA for isolated tibial side loosening; 14 experienced an isolated tibial component revision (isolated cohort), and 17 experienced total (both femoral and tibial components) revision surgery (total cohort). The postoperative ROM, Western Ontario and McMaster Universities Arthritis (WOMAC) index, KSKS, KSFS, and mechanical axis (MA) were compared between the two cohorts. The intraoperative tourniquet time and amount of blood drainage were also compared. The mean follow-up durations in the isolated and total cohorts were 40.7 and 56.1 months, respectively. Both cohorts had similar postoperative ROM, WOMAC index, KSKS, KSFS, and MA; however, substantially shorter tourniquet time (105.2 versus 154.6 min) and less blood drainage (417.2 versus 968.1 mL) were found in the isolated cohort than in the total cohort. Isolated tibial component rTKA for tibial component loosening exhibited comparable clinical and radiological results to those of total rTKA. The pros of the isolated tibial component revision surgery were short operation time and small blood loss [8].

In a study with level 3 of evidence published in 2023, Apinyankul et al. compared isolated versus full-component revision in TKA for aseptic loosening [1]. Between January 2009 and December 2019, a consecutive cohort of revision TKA was reviewed. Univariate and multivariable analyses were utilized to study correlations among factors and surgical related adverse events, time to prosthesis failure, and functional results (University of California Los Angeles (UCLA), KSSF, knee osteoarthritis and outcome score for joint replacement (KOOS-JR), Veterans RAND 12 (VR-12) physical, and VR-12 mental). A total of 238 individuals experienced rTKA for aseptic loosening. The mean follow-up time was 5 years (range 25–152 months). Ten of the 105 individuals (9.5%) who experienced full revision (both femoral and tibial components) and 18 of the 133 (13.5%) who experienced isolated revision had subsequent prosthesis failure (Fig. 6.2). The factor analysis of type of revision (full or isolated revision) did not show a substantial difference between cohorts in terms of adverse events, implant failures, and times to failure. Metallosis was related to early time to failure and iliotibial band release was

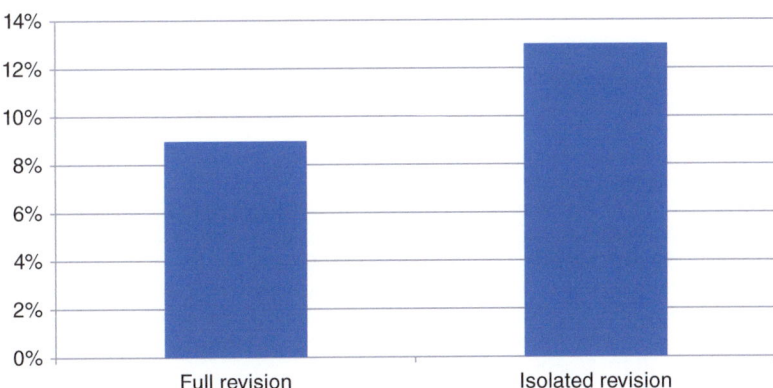

Fig. 6.2 Isolated versus full-component revision in total knee arthroplasty (TKA) for aseptic loosening: rates of subsequent prosthesis failure [1]

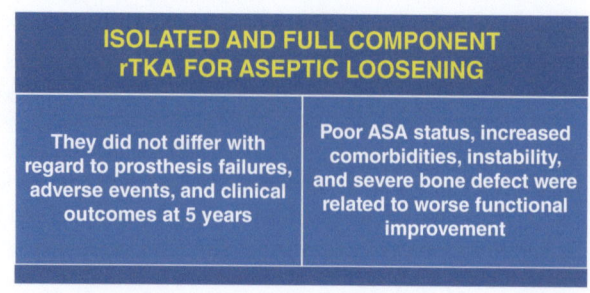

Fig. 6.3 Isolated versus full-component revision in total knee arthroplasty (TKA) for aseptic loosening: summary of the conclusions of the study of Apinyankul et al. [1]. rTKA = revision total knee arthroplasty; ASA = American Society of Anesthesiologists

associated with more adverse events. Preoperative symptoms of instability were associated with the worst improvement in UCLA score. Higher American Society of Anesthesiologists (ASA) status and higher Charlson Comorbidity Index (CCI) were related with worse VR-12 physical (−30.5) and KOOS-JR (−4.2) scores, respectively. The main conclusions of this study are summarized in Fig. 6.3 [1].

6.4 Conclusions

ITPIE seems to be a dependable treatment for instability and/or PE wear following TKA in the presence of well-fixed and well-aligned components with good survival and clinical improvement. The less invasive nature and diminished risk for bone loss made it an attractive alternative versus full revision. Regarding partial-component versus full-component rTKA, isolated and full-component rTKA for aseptic loosening did not differ with respect to prosthesis failures, adverse events, and clinical outcomes at 5 years. Poor ASA status, increased comorbidities, instability, and a severe bone defect were related to worse functional improvement.

References

1. Apinyankul R, Hwang K, Segovia NA, Amanatullah DF, Huddleston JI, Maloney WJ, et al. Isolated versus full component revision in total knee arthroplasty for aseptic loosening. J Arthroplast. 2023;38(2):335–40. https://doi.org/10.1016/j.arth.2022.09.006.
2. Babis GC, Trousdale RT, Morrey BF. The effectiveness of isolated tibial insert exchange in revision total knee arthroplasty. J Bone Joint Surg Am. 2002;84(1):64–8. https://doi.org/10.2106/00004623-200201000-00010.
3. Willson SE, Munro ML, Sandwell JC, Ezzet KA, Colwell CW Jr. Isolated tibial polyethylene insert exchange outcomes after total knee arthroplasty. Clin Orthop Relat Res. 2010;468(1):96–101. https://doi.org/10.1007/s11999-009-1023-3.
4. Cooper HJ, Moya-Angeler J, Bas-Aguilar MA, Hepinstall MS, Scuderi GR, Rodriguez J. Isolated polyethylene exchange with increased constraint is comparable to component revision TKA for instability in properly selected patients. J Arthroplast. 2018;33(9):2946–51. https://doi.org/10.1016/j.arth.2018.04.042.
5. Tetreault MW, Hines JT, Berry DJ, Pagnano MW, Trousdale RT, Abdel MP. Isolated tibial insert exchange in revision total knee arthroplasty: reliable and durable for wear; less so for

instability, insert fracture/dissociation, or stiffness. Bone Joint J. 2021;103-B(6):1103–10. https://doi.org/10.1302/0301-620X.103B6.BJJ-2020-1954.R2.
6. Alexander JS, Richardson E, Crawford DA, Berend KR, Morris MJ, Lombardi AV Jr. Isolated tibial polyethylene insert exchange after total knee arthroplasty for treatment of instability and/or polyethylene wear. Surg Technol Int. 2022;42:sti42/1654. https://doi.org/10.52198/23.STI.42.OS1654. Online ahead of print.
7. Fehring TK, Odum S, Griffin WL, Mason JB. Outcome comparison of partial and full component revision TKA. Clin Orthop Relat Res. 2005;440:131–4. https://doi.org/10.1097/01.blo.0000186560.70566.dc.
8. Lee SS, Park JS, Lee YK, Moon YW. Comparison of the clinical and radiological outcomes between an isolated tibial component revision and total revision knee arthroplasty in aseptic loosening of an isolated tibial component. J Orthop Sci. 2021;26(3):435–40. https://doi.org/10.1016/j.jos.2020.05.007.

Wound Complications Following Revision Total Knee Arthroplasty

7

E. Carlos Rodríguez-Merchán, Carlos A. Encinas-Ullán, Juan S. Ruiz-Pérez, and Primitivo Gómez-Cardero

7.1 Introduction

Wound healing in revision total knee arthroplasty (rTKA) can be jeopardized due to increased surgical dissection and poorer soft tissue quality and vascularity from previous surgical procedures [1, 2]. However, there are limited data on the final clinical course of these individuals. The purpose of this chapter is to review the prevalence of wound complications in rTKA, factors that increase the risk of wound complications, and the results of rTKA following development of wound complications.

7.2 Prevalence

In 2016, Belmont et al. analyzed the readmissions after rTKA in the National Surgical Quality Improvement Program database and encountered a readmission rate of 1% and 0.4% for superficial and wound disruptions, respectively [3]. Development of a wound complication without deep infection following rTKA increased the reoperations but did not lead to a substantial increase of subsequent resection arthroplasties in both aseptic and reimplantation individuals [4].

In 2019, Carter et al. stated that wound complications were the most common early adverse event after rTKA with 0.5% individuals needing return to the operating room [5]. In 2019, Petis et al. reported that wound healing problems were the most common adverse event after rTKA in a series of 245 individuals. Nine (3.7%) needed return to the operating room for wound debridement and closure [6]. In

---

E. C. Rodríguez-Merchán (✉) · C. A. Encinas-Ullán · J. S. Ruiz-Pérez · P. Gómez-Cardero
Department of Orthopedic Surgery, La Paz University Hospital, Madrid, Spain

© The Author(s), under exclusive license to Springer Nature Switzerland AG 2024
E. C. Rodríguez-Merchán (ed.), *Advances in Revision Total Knee Arthroplasty*,
https://doi.org/10.1007/978-3-031-60445-4_7

2023, Koressel et al. reported a 2.4% rate of return to the operating room for a wound complication after rTKA (1.8% wound complication rate for aseptic rTKA) [7].

7.3 Preventive Measures and Treatment

Wound problems are a feared adverse event after total knee arthroplasty (TKA) and the goal is to prevent them. Preventive measures are shown in Fig. 7.1. Should continuous wound drainage or soft tissue necrosis happen, prompt intervention is mandatory, because postponement risks deep infection and failure of the TKA. Cases associated with full-thickness soft tissue necrosis frequently need transfer of well-vascularized tissue, such as a medial gastrocnemius myocutaneous flap reconstruction [8].

According to Vince and Abdeen, wound problems can frequently be averted with attentive planning. When transverse incisions are utilized for knee surgery many years prior to any anticipated knee arthroplasty, no major problems are typically found with a conventional, anterior longitudinal incision. They advised lateral incisions (e.g., after a prior lateral tibial plateau fracture) be reutilized for TKA. When faced with many prior incisions, surgeons would best utilize the most recently healed or the most lateral. Vince and Abdeen favor soft tissue reconstruction with expanders or a gastrocnemius flap if there are many incisions, if the skin and scar tissue are adherent to underlying tissue, or if wound healing appears doubtful. Deep infection should be confirmed by aspiration. When present, treatment should include irrigation, débridement, polyethylene exchange if acute, and resection arthroplasty if chronic. Poor wound healing is a potentially calamitous adverse event that might lead to many reconstructive procedures and even amputation. Prompt identification followed by expeditious débridement and soft tissue reconstruction should be utilized for treating wound complications following TKA [9].

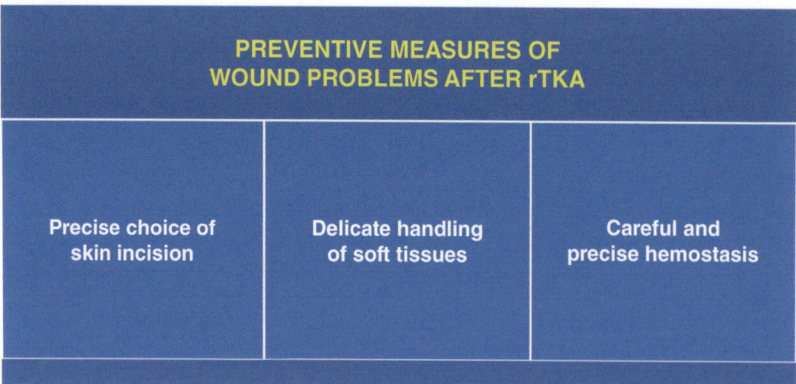

Fig. 7.1 Preventive measures of wound problems after revision total knee arthroplasty (rTKA)

In 2011, Garbedian et al. stated that it was paramount not to underestimate the significance of wound complications after TKA. Appropriate and aggressive care was advised. Comprehending the blood supply to the skin around the knee and measures to avert wound complications are essential to avoiding wound problems. A detailed patient history and physical examination will recognize high-risk individuals and any modifiable risk factors. Operative techniques such as raising full-thickness skin flaps and wise placement of skin incisions in the presence of previous scars can significantly diminish the prevalence of wound problems. The first step in managing wound problems is identifying when a problem is present and knowing when a minor problem can transform into a major one. Superficial infections or stitch abscesses can be managed with conservative treatment. Nonetheless, the surgeon should have a low threshold to return to surgical treatment if drainage lingers. Skin necrosis or nonviable skin should be excised in the operating room, and the existence of a deep infection must be diagnosed by joint aspiration. The adequate course of action in handling deep infection depends on the duration elapsed since the index procedure. The capacity to carry out a medial gastrocnemius muscle flap and skin graft is a valuable ability in complicated cases where primary wound closure cannot be accomplished. Careful and precise attention to detail during surgery and aggressive surgical management of wound complications can be the difference in saving the knee [10].

According to Sharma et al., advanced dressings such as film and Hydrofiber dressings have fewer wound adverse events and better fluid handling ability, but insufficient evidence is accessible to know whether the utilization of these advanced dressings diminish periprosthetic joint infection (PJI) [11]. The optimal management of wounds after rTKA endures undetermined. Negative pressure wound therapy (NPWT) has been demonstrated efficacious in reducing wound complications in rTKAs. Higuera et al. demonstrated that NPWT reduced the percentages of surgical site infections (SSIs) in a randomized controlled trial after rTKA [12]. Newman et al. also published that reoperations in individuals after rTKA treated with NPWT were also substantially reduced compared to controls [13].

According to Colen et al., it seems that with adequate treatment, many wound complications can be salvaged with timely and appropriate surgical intervention. Prompt participation of plastic surgeons to manage the soft tissue envelope may diminish management failures and subsequent procedures with ever increasing risk of infection and failures [4].

7.4 Conditions Associated with an Increased Risk for Wound Complications After rTKA

7.4.1 Atrial Fibrillation

Atrial fibrillation has been found to be independently associated with wound complications when both aseptic revisions and reimplantations were combined [7].

7.4.2 Connective Tissue Disorders

Individuals with connective tissue diseases can have impaired wound healing and hematoma formation after surgery [14]. According to Koressel et al., connective tissue condition was a risk factor for the development of wound complication within the aseptic revision cohort, while a history of depression was associated with the development of wound complication within the reimplantation cohort [7].

7.4.3 Vasculitis

Vasculitis that impairs the microcirculation of the subcutaneous tissues but also the combination that some of these individuals need immunomodulating drugs to manage their diseases and stronger postoperative anticoagulation might also play roles in impaired wound healing [15].

7.4.4 Body Mass Index, Smoking Status, and Diabetes

Body mass index (BMI), smoking status, and a diagnosis of diabetes have been demonstrated to predispose the individuals to wound healing problems after rTKA [16, 17].

7.5 Outcomes

In 2023, Koressel et al. analyzed 585 rTKAs with 2-year follow-up carried out between 2012 and 2019 [7]. The indication for rTKA included aseptic etiologies (i.e., loosening, instability, stiffness) and individuals who successfully completed antibiotic treatment after resection arthroplasty as part of a two-stage exchange protocol. Wound closure methods for rTKA were variable and at the surgeon's discretion. In general, aseptic revisions were closed utilizing skin staples, while individuals experiencing subsequent two-stage reimplantation were closed utilizing sutures in a mattress fashion. In some instances, negative pressure wound dressings were applied, and most individuals were immobilized for a minimum period of 7 days. The majority if patients received aspirin for deep venous thrombosis (DVT) prophylaxis. Individuals experiencing irrigation, debridement, and modular component exchanges for acute infection (DAIR) as well as those individuals with persistent infection managed with antibiotic spacer exchange, knee arthrodesis, and amputation were excluded from the study. There were 399 aseptic revisions and 186 reimplantation rTKA following treatment for PJI. There were 376 men and 209 women with a mean age of 62 years. The wound complication cohort included only individuals with a superficial wound complication without deep infection needing return to the operating room within 120 days. A superficial wound complication was defined as dehiscence, persistent drainage, skin necrosis, superficial infection, or deferred wound healing without proof of violation of the deep fascia seen at the time of surgery. All individuals experienced irrigation and debridement with or without additional plastic surgery intervention. An extensile approach to the knee was utilized in order to confirm the integrity of the arthrotomy. In cases in which an aspiration was not carried out preoperatively, an intraoperative joint aspiration after superficial debridement was carried out to confirm the absence of a deep joint infection [7].

The results for the aseptic rTKA cohort were analyzed separately from those experiencing rTKA as part of reimplantation for management of PJI to minimize confounding due to differences in infection among the two cohorts. Host factors, rates of subsequent deep infection, and reoperations and re-rTKA of rTKA were compared between individuals with and without superficial wound complication needing reoperation after rTKA within each cohort only. The mean follow-up in this cohort of individuals experiencing rTKA was 49.2 months. There were no substantial differences in patient demographics and comorbidities in individuals experiencing aseptic rTKA compared to those experiencing rTKA for reimplantation. 2% individuals who experienced aseptic rTKA developed a wound complication without deep infection compared to 4% individuals experiencing revision as part of their two-stage reimplantation procedure (Fig. 7.2). The mean time to return to the operating room was 35.6 days versus 28.3 days in individuals experiencing aseptic rTKA and reimplantation TKA, respectively. The development of superficial wound complication after rTKA increased the risk for subsequent deep infection in individuals experiencing aseptic rTKA but did not have the same impact in individuals experiencing reimplantation TKA. Overall, the rates of subsequent development of deep infection were 4% in the aseptic revision cohort compared to 21% in the reimplantation cohort at last follow-up (Fig. 7.3). Individuals experiencing aseptic rTKA who developed a wound complication needing surgical intervention were ten times

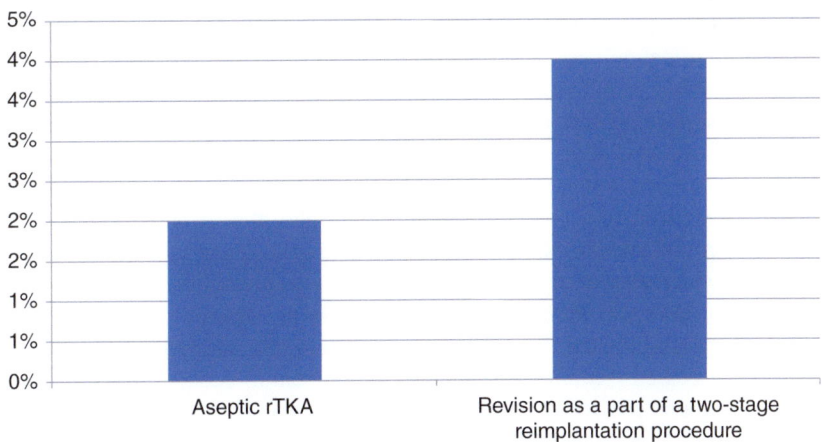

Fig. 7.2 Rates of a wound complication without deep infection after revision total knee arthroplasty (rTKA)

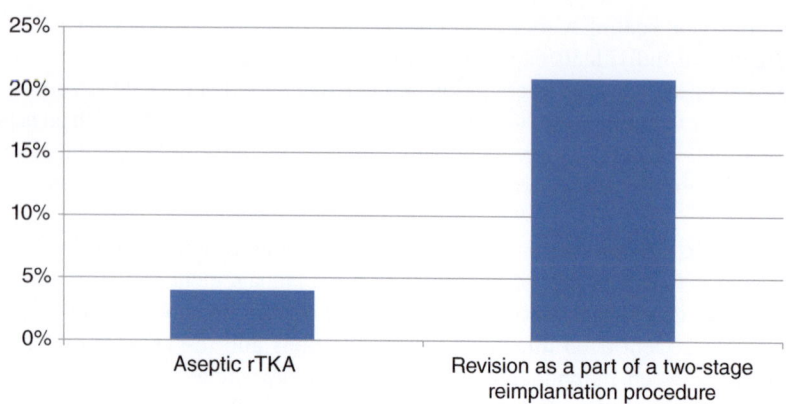

Fig. 7.3 Rates of subsequent development of deep infection after superficial wound complication following revision total knee arthroplasty (rTKA)

more likely to develop a subsequent deep infection compared to individuals without wound complications. In contrast, individuals experiencing reimplantation TKA with a wound complication were not at a substantially increased risk of developing a subsequent deep infection compared to controls. The mean time to reinfection in the setting of a wound complication was 290.2 days after index revision compared 546 days in those who did not develop a wound complication. Multivariate regression analysis identified a few conditions associated with an increased risk for wound complications after rTKA [7].

A wound complication after aseptic rTKA was associated with increased reoperations (2.1 versus 0.2) but not eventual removal of implants compared to controls. In individuals experiencing reimplantation TKA, a wound complication also increased the risk of reoperations (3.3 versus 0.7) but not eventual resection arthroplasty compared to those who did not develop a wound problem. Individuals experiencing rTKA were at increased risk for development of wound complications without deep infection needing reoperation compared to primary TKA individuals (2.4% prevalence). In individuals experiencing both component revision for aseptic etiologies, the development of a wound complication without deep infection needing return to the operating room significantly increased the risk for subsequent PJI. This association was not found in individuals experiencing rTKA as part of a two-stage reimplantation procedure which highlights that a previous history of infection might be the most significant predictor of subsequent infection. The reoperations were increased after the development of a wound complication, but the risk of subsequent resection arthroplasty was not different compared to their controls. These findings highlighted the importance of timely and adequate intervention as well as the increased risk of development of subsequent infections among individuals experiencing rTKA for all causes [7]. Figure 7.4 shows a case of chronic infections after TKA. Figures 7.5 and 7.6 show two cases of chronic infection after TKA and their treatment.

Fig. 7.4 Chronic infection after total knee arthroplasty (TKA)

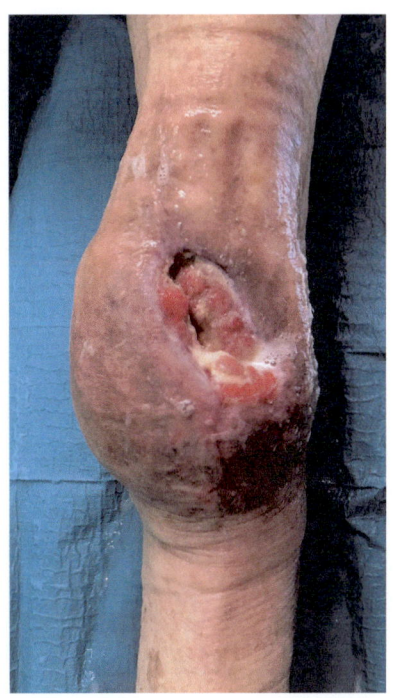

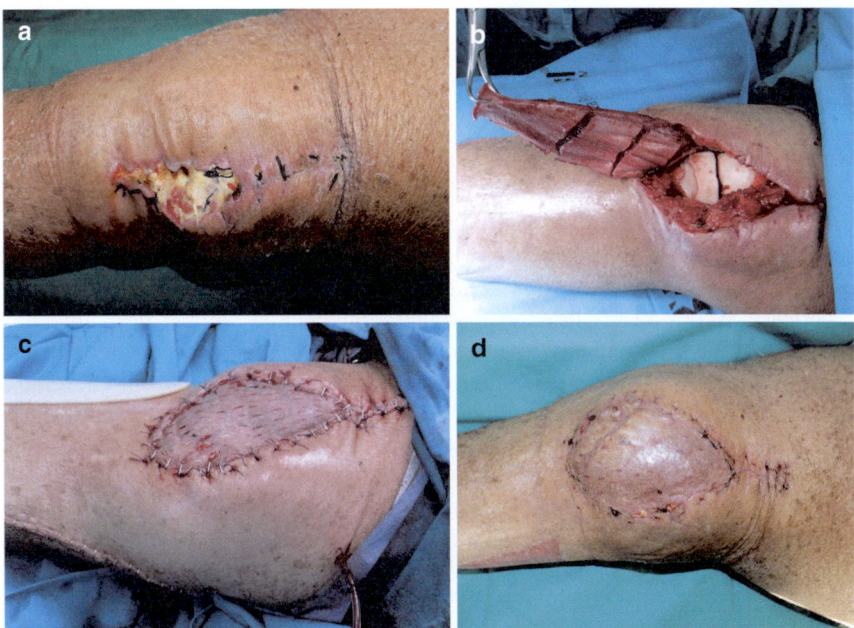

Fig. 7.5 (**a–d**) Chronic infection after total knee arthroplasty (TKA) (**a**); medial gastrocnemius graft flap (**b**); mesh skin graft (**c**); one month after surgery (**d**)

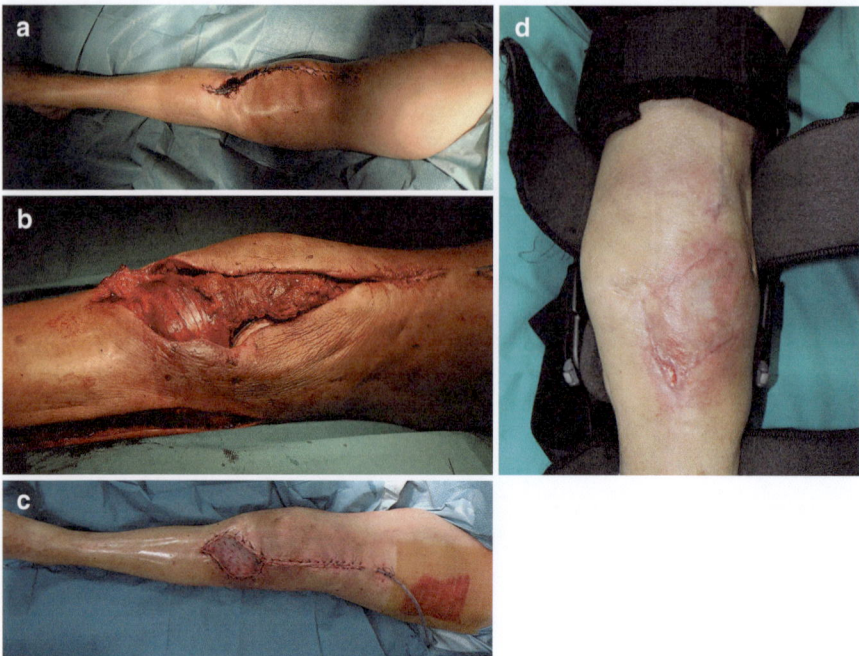

Fig. 7.6 (**a–d**) Necrotic area in the surgical wound after total knee arthroplasty (TKA) (**a**); lateral gastrocnemius flap (**b**); mesh skin graft (**c**); 3 months after surgery (**d**)

7.6   Conclusions

Wound complications needing return to the operating room for wound debridement and closure after rTKA occur in 0.5–3.7% individuals. Prevention of wound problems is paramount. Preventive measures include precise choice of the skin incision, delicate handling of the soft tissues, careful and precise hemostasis, and wound closure without excessive tension. It has been published that 1.8% individuals who experience aseptic rTKA develop a wound complication without deep infection compared to 3.8% individuals experiencing rTKA as part of a two-stage reimplantation procedure. Also, those individuals experiencing aseptic rTKA who develop a wound complication needing surgical intervention are ten times more likely to develop a subsequent deep infection compared to individuals without wound complications. Wound complications following rTKA are potentially calamitous adverse events that might lead to many reconstructive procedures and even amputation. Prompt identification followed by expeditious débridement and soft tissue reconstruction should be utilized.

References

1. Osei DA, Rebehn KA, Boyer MI. Soft-tissue defects after total knee arthroplasty: management and reconstruction. J Am Acad Orthop Surg. 2016;24(11):769–79. https://doi.org/10.5435/JAAOS-D-15-00241.
2. Lee GC, Colen DL, Levin LS, Kovach SJ. Microvascular free flap coverage for salvage of the infected total knee arthroplasty: a triumph of technique over reason? Bone Joint J. 2020;102-B(6_Supple_A):176–80. https://doi.org/10.1302/0301-620X.102B6.BJJ-2019-1661.R1.
3. Belmont PJ, Goodman GP, Rodriguez M, Bader JO, Waterman BR, Schoenfeld AJ. Predictors of hospital readmission following revision total knee arthroplasty. Knee Surg Sports Traumatol Arthrosc. 2016;24(10):3329–38. https://doi.org/10.1007/s00167-015-3782-6.
4. Colen DL, Carney MJ, Shubinets V, Lanni MA, Liu TBS, Scott Levin L, et al. Soft-tissue reconstruction of the complicated knee arthroplasty: principles and predictors of salvage. Plast Reconstr Surg. 2018;141(4):1040–8. https://doi.org/10.1097/PRS.0000000000004255.
5. Carter J, Springer B, Curtin BM. Early complications of revision total knee arthroplasty in morbidly obese patients. Eur J Orthop Surg Traumatol. 2019;29(5):1101–4. https://doi.org/10.1007/s00590-019-02403-9.
6. Petis SM, Perry KI, Mabry TM, Hanssen AD, Berry DJ, Abdel MP. Two-stage exchange protocol for periprosthetic joint infection following total knee arthroplasty in 245 knees without prior treatment for infection. J Bone Joint Surg Am. 2019;101(3):239–49. https://doi.org/10.2106/JBJS.18.00356.
7. Koressel J, Perez BA, Minutillo GT, Granruth CB, Mastrangelo S, Lee GC. Wound complications following revision total knee arthroplasty: prevalence and outcomes. Knee. 2023;42:44–50. https://doi.org/10.1016/j.knee.2023.02.011.
8. Dennis DA. Wound complications in total knee arthroplasty. Instr Course Lect. 1997;46:165–9.
9. Vince KG, Abdeen A. Wound problems in total knee arthroplasty. Clin Orthop Relat Res. 2006;452:88–90. https://doi.org/10.1097/01.blo.0000238821.71271.cc.
10. Garbedian S, Sternheim A, Backstein D. Wound healing problems in total knee arthroplasty. Orthopedics. 2011;34(9):e516–8. https://doi.org/10.3928/01477447-20110714-42.
11. Sharma G, Lee SW, Atanacio O, Parvizi J, Kim TK. In search of the optimal wound dressing material following total hip and knee arthroplasty: a systematic review and meta-analysis. Int Orthop. 2017;41(7):1295–305. https://doi.org/10.1007/s00264-017-3484-4.
12. Higuera-Rueda CA, Emara AK, Nieves-Malloure Y, Klika AK, Cooper HJ, Cross MB, et al. The effectiveness of closed-incision negative-pressure therapy versus silver-impregnated dressings in mitigating surgical site complications in high-risk patients after revision knee arthroplasty: the PROMISES randomized controlled trial. J Arthroplasty. 2021;36(7S):S295–S302.e14. https://doi.org/10.1016/j.arth.2021.02.076.
13. Newman JM, Siqueira MBP, Klika AK, Molloy RM, Barsoum WK, Higuera CA. Use of closed incisional negative pressure wound therapy after revision total hip and knee arthroplasty in patients at high risk for infection: a prospective, randomized clinical trial. J Arthroplasty. 2019;34(3):554–559.e1. https://doi.org/10.1016/j.arth.2018.11.017.
14. Rubio GA, Mundra LS, Thaller SR. Association of autoimmune connective tissue disease with abdominoplasty outcomes: a nationwide analysis of outcomes. JAMA Surg. 2018;153(2):186–8. https://doi.org/10.1001/jamasurg.2017.3796.
15. Guo S, DiPietro LA. Critical review in oral biology & medicine: factors affecting wound healing. J Dent Res. 2010;89(3):219–29. https://doi.org/10.1177/0022034509359125.
16. Sørensen LT, Hemmingsen U, Kallehave F, Wille-Jørgensen P, Kjærgaard J, Møller LN, et al. Risk factors for tissue and wound complications in gastrointestinal surgery. Ann Surg. 2005;241(4):654–8. https://doi.org/10.1097/01.sla.0000157131.84130.12.
17. Carroll K, Dowsey M, Choong P, Peel T. Risk factors for superficial wound complications in hip and knee arthroplasty. Clin Microbiol Infect. 2014;20(2):130–5. https://doi.org/10.1111/1469-0691.12209.

One-Stage Revision Total Knee Arthroplasty for Periprosthetic Joint Infection

8

E. Carlos Rodríguez-Merchán, Carlos A. Encinas-Ullán, Juan S. Ruiz-Pérez, and Primitivo Gómez-Cardero

8.1 Introduction

Total knee arthroplasty (TKA) is turning into an ordinary surgical procedure in orthopedic surgery. One of the plausible adverse events of this surgery is periprosthetic joint infection (PJI) [1]. PJI of the knee represents a severe complication after 1.5–2% of primary TKAs [2]. Revision TKA (rTKA) is challenging to carry out in individuals with PJI because of the difficulty of eliminating the infection and possibility for osseous and ligamentous deficits [3]. According to Raziie et al., two-stage revision has traditionally been contemplated the gold standard of treatment for proven infection, but growing proof is coming out in support of one-stage exchange for selected individuals [4].

In 2023, Wignadasan et al. stated that a PJI was possibly the most significant potential adverse event of TKA and was associated with significant morbidity and socioeconomic burden. It is a disastrous adverse event for both the patient and the orthopedic surgeon alike. A two-stage revision strategy for infected TKA has been the standard for surgical management; however, there is growing interest in single-stage revision surgery due to fewer procedures, diminished inpatient hospital stay, and diminished expenses to healthcare systems. The two-stage strategy implies the employment of an antibiotic spacer prior to the second stage is performed. Individuals with a PJI should be managed by a multidisciplinary team. These individuals should be treated in specialist arthroplasty centers by high volume revision arthroplasty specialists [5].

PJIs with previous numerous failed surgeries for reinfection constitute an enormous defiance for surgeons due to bad vascular supply and biofilm formation [6]. The objective of this chapter is to analyze the outcomes of single-stage rTKA for PJI.

E. C. Rodríguez-Merchán (✉) · C. A. Encinas-Ullán · J. S. Ruiz-Pérez · P. Gómez-Cardero
Department of Orthopedic Surgery, La Paz University Hospital, Madrid, Spain

© The Author(s), under exclusive license to Springer Nature Switzerland AG 2024
E. C. Rodríguez-Merchán (ed.), *Advances in Revision Total Knee Arthroplasty*,
https://doi.org/10.1007/978-3-031-60445-4_8

8.2 Indications for a Single-Stage rTKA

In 2019, Thakrar et al. performed a systematic review of the literature with the objective of proposing criteria for the selection of individuals for a single-stage exchange arthroplasty in the treatment of a PJI. They concluded that single-stage revision was an acceptable form of surgical treatment for the management of a PJI in selected individuals. The indications for this technique included the absence of serious immunocompromise and substantial soft tissue or osseous compromise and coexisting acute sepsis. They advised that a two-stage approach should be utilized in individuals with multidrug-resistant or atypical organisms such as fungus [7].

According to Wignadasan et al., one-stage exchange is indicated when there is no sign of systemic sepsis and in cases where a microorganism has been isolated. It involves removal of the old prosthesis, debridement of all infected tissue, a copious washout and redraping, and finally, reimplantation of a new prosthesis [5]. Figures 8.1 and 8.2 show a case of chronic infection in TKA treated by means of one-stage revision arthroplasty of the femoral component and Bactisure Wound Lavage (Zimmer Biomet Solution with ethanol, acetic acid, sodium acetate) in *Streptococcus mitis* infection.

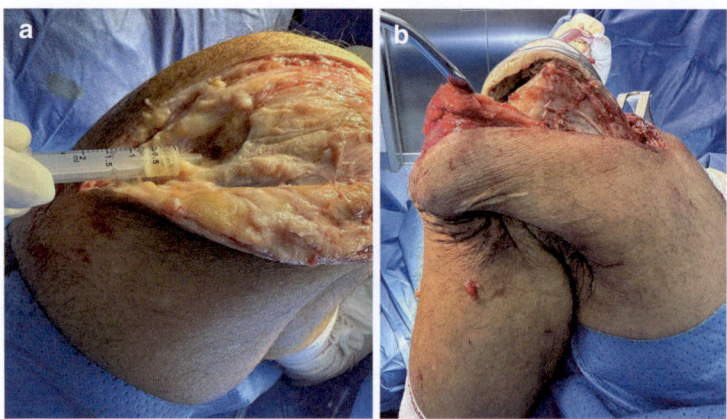

Fig. 8.1 (**a**, **b**) Chronic infection in total knee arthroplasty (**a**); severe osteolysis and septic loosening of femoral component (**b**)

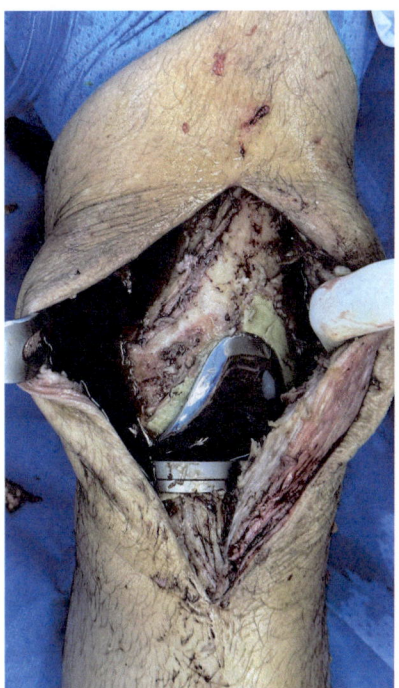

Fig. 8.2 One-stage revision of the femoral component and Bactisure wound lavage (Zimmer Biomet Solution with ethanol, acetic acid, sodium acetate) in *Streptococcus mitis* infection

8.3 Antibiotic Prophylaxis in One-Stage Revision of Septic TKA

In a scoping review published in 2023 by Ciccullo et al., they studied which antibiotic is employed as prophylaxis for septic one-stage rTKA and what is the rationale for its employment. They found no article capable of responding the question of which antibiotic to employ as surgical prophylaxis for a septic one-stage rTKA. They advised employing the same antibiotic prophylaxis as for primary TKA, i.e., cefazolin (for its low side effect percentage and relative efficacy) [1].

8.4 Outcomes of Single-Stage rTKA for Periprosthetic Joint Infection

8.4.1 Comparable Clinical Results of Culture-Negative and Culture-Positive PJIs

In a systematic review published in 2023 by Li et al., they compared the clinical results of culture-negative PJI (CN PJI) with those of culture-positive PJI (CP PJI) [8]. The pooled outcomes of the included studies exhibited that overall failure rate in CN PJI cohort (19%) was substantially inferior than that in CP PJI cohort (23.4%).

They carried out the subgroup analysis based on the surgical strategies, the pooled outcomes of nine studies for individuals experiencing debridement, antibiotics, and implant retention (DAIR) showed that failure rate in CN PJI cohort (22.2%) was substantially inferior than that in CP PJI cohort (29.3%), the pooled outcomes of four studies for individuals experiencing one-stage revision showed that failure rate between CN PJI cohort (11.5%) and CP PJI cohort (7.6%) had no substantial difference, and the pooled outcomes of 19 studies for individuals experiencing two-stage revision showed that failure rate in CN PJI cohort (16.1%) was substantially inferior than that in CP PJI cohort (20.4%). CN PJI cohort had similar or better survival percentage when compared with CP PJI cohort for individuals who experienced DAIR (debridement, antibiotics, and implant retention), one-stage revision, or two-stage revision. Negative culture was not a worse prognostic factor for PJI [8].

8.4.2 Midterm Results

In 2021, Razii et al. analyzed the outcomes of single-stage rTKA for PJI, with mid-run follow-up [4]. A total of 84 individuals, with a mean age of 68 years, experienced single-stage rTKA for proven PJI between 2006 and 2016. In all, 37 individuals (44%) were treated for an infected primary TKA (pTKA), while the majority presented with infected revisions: 31 had experienced one previous revision (36.9%) and 16 had multiple prior revisions (19.1%). Contraindications to the procedure were systemic sepsis, large osseous or soft tissue loss, extensor mechanism failure, or if primary wound closure was improbable to be obtainable. Individuals were not excluded for culture-negative PJI or the presence of a sinus. Overall, 76 individuals (90.5%) were infection-free at a mean follow-up of 7 years, with eight reinfections (9.5%). Culture-negative PJI was not associated with a higher reinfection percentage. However, there was a substantially higher percentage of recurrence in individuals with polymicrobial infections. The mean Oxford Knee Score (OKS) improved from 18.7 before surgery to 33.8 at 6 months after surgery. The Kaplan-Meier implant survival rate for all causes of reoperation, including reinfection and aseptic failure, was 95.2% at 1 year, 83.5% at 5 years, and 78.9% at 12 years. One-stage exchange, utilizing a strict debridement protocol and multidisciplinary advice, was an efficacious management alternative for the infected TKA [4].

8.4.3 Reinfection Percentage, Infection-Free Survival Following Reoperation for Recurrent Infection, and the Pathogens Implicated in Both Primary and Recurrent Infection

In a systematic review with level 4 of evidence published in 2023 by Bosco et al., they evaluated reinfection percentage, infection-free survival after reoperation for recurrent infection, and the pathogens implicated in both primary and recurrent infection [2]. A reinfection rate of 12.2% after an average follow-up of 57.6 months was found. The most common causative pathogens were gram-positive bacteria (71.1%), gram-negative bacteria (7.1%), and polymicrobial infections (8%). The infection-free survival following management for repeating infection was 92.1%. The causative pathogens at reinfections differed substantially from the primary infection (gram-positive 44.4%, gram-negative 11.1%). Individuals who experienced a one-stage rTKA for PJI exhibited a reinfection percentage inferior or comparable to other surgical treatments as two-stage or DAIR. Reoperation for reinfection showed an inferior success compared to one-stage rTKA. Furthermore, microbiology differed between primary infection and repeating infection [2].

8.4.4 One-Stage rTKA for Enterococcal Periprosthetic Joint Infection

In 2021, Rossmann et al. affirmed that a wide range of success rates after surgical management of enterococcal PJI with a tendency toward worse results had been reported. However, the role of one-stage exchange remained unclear [9]. They assessed their outcomes following the one-stage knee exchange for enterococcal PJI. Forty individuals were retrospectively included between 2002 and 2017 with a mean follow-up of survivors of 80 months (range 22–172). Polymicrobial infections happened in 45% (18/40) of individuals. Revision surgery was needed in 22 cases (55%) with a mean time to revision surgery of 27 months (range 1–78). Indications for aseptic revisions (18%) included aseptic loosening (10%), periprosthetic fracture (5%), and patellar instability (3%). The most frequent cause of re-revision was a subsequent PJI (15/22; 68%) after a mean time of 22 months (range 1–77). Overall infection recurrence rate was 37.5% (15/40), significantly due to entirely nonenterococcal infections (9/15; 60%). Infection relapse with *Enterococci* happened in four cases (10%) within 16 months postoperatively. Older individuals and male gender were related to a higher risk of infection recurrence. Overcoming the *Enterococci* utilizing the one-stage exchange for knee PJI is feasible, but the percentage of reinfection due to new microorganisms is high. However, the overall infection recurrence percentage was comparable to other treatment strategies [9].

8.4.5 Infected Rotating-Hinge Implants Treated with One-Stage-Exchange: Midterm Survivorship

In a study with level 4 of evidence published in 2021, Ohlmeier et al. stated that in spite of the growing number of studies reporting on PJI, there were little data on one-stage exchange arthroplasty for the revision of infected rotating-hinge prostheses, which can be among the most challenging PJI presentations to manage [10]. After one-stage direct exchange revision for an infected rotating-hinge TKA prosthesis, and utilizing a multimodal strategy for infection control, Ohlmeier et al. analyzed the survivorship free from repeat revision for infection and survivorship free from reoperation for any cause and the clinical result, based on the OKS, of these individuals at the latest follow-up. Between January 2011 and December 2017, they treated 101 individuals with infected rotating-hinge knee prostheses. All individuals who experienced a one-stage exchange utilizing another rotating-hinge implant were potentially eligible for the study. During that period, they generally utilized a one-stage strategy when managing PJIs. Eighty-three percent (84 of 101) of individuals were treated with one-stage exchange, and 17% (17 of 1001) were treated with two-stage exchange. Of the 84 treated with one-stage exchange, eight individuals died of unrelated causes and were therefore excluded, one individual refused to take part in the study, and another eight individuals were lost before the minimum study follow-up of 2 years or had incomplete datasets, leaving 80% (67 of 84) for analysis. The included study population consisted of 60% men (40 of 67) with a mean age of 64 years and a mean body mass index (BMI) of 30 kg/m^2. The mean number of previous surgeries was four on the affected knee. Fifteen percent (10 of 67) of knees had a preoperative joint communicating sinus tract, and 66% (44 of 67) had undergone a previous PJI on the affected knee. The mean follow-up duration was 6 years. Kaplan-Meier survivorship analysis was carried out utilizing the end points of survivorship free from repeat revision for infection and survivorship free from all-cause revision. The functional result was evaluated utilizing the OKS (on a 12- to 60-point scale, with lower scores representing less pain and greater function), attained by interviewing individuals for this study at their most recent follow-up visit. The Kaplan-Meier analysis showed an overall survivorship free from reoperation for any cause of 75% at the mean follow-up of 6 years postoperatively. Survivorship free from any repeat operative procedure for infection was 90% at 6 years. The mean postoperative OKS was 37 points. With an overall revision percentage of around 25% at 6 years and the limited functional outcomes based on the poor OKSs, individuals should be counseled to have modest expectations concerning postoperative pain and function level after one-stage exchange of an infected rotating-hinge arthroplasty. Nonetheless, individuals may be notified about a modest possibility of PJI elimination and may opt for this strategy as a means to try to avert high transfemoral amputation or joint arthrodesis, which in these individuals frequently is associated with the incapacity to ambulate at all [10].

8.4.6 Results of One-Stage rTKA in Terms of Eradication of the Infection, Improvement of Pain, and Knee Function

In 2021, Pellegrini et al. assessed the results of one-stage rTKA in terms of eradication of the infection, improvement of pain, and knee function [11]. Between 2009 and 2016, 20 individuals experienced one-stage rTKA for the treatment of a PJI. Inclusion criteria were individuals non-immunocompromised with minimal or moderate bone loss, known organisms with known sensitivity. Evaluation included clinical signs of infection eradication, range of motion (ROM), Knee Society (KS) clinical rating score, visual analog scale (VAS) pain score, and radiographic evaluation. After a mean follow-up of 6.2 years (range, 2–10 years), none of the individuals had signs suggesting recurrent infection. Follow-up examination demonstrated substantial improvement of all variables compared to preoperative values. One-stage revision surgery rendered infection eradication and satisfying subjective functional results for infected knee arthroplasty in selected individuals. One-stage rTKA was a helpful technique to approach PJIs in selected individuals whose infecting microorganism and sensitivity are determined prior to surgery. In order to be successful, strict inclusion criteria should be applied, as only non-immunocompromised individuals with healthy soft tissues with minimal or moderate bone loss are eligible for this surgical technique [11].

8.4.7 One-Stage rTKA for PJI: The Clinical Result of Different TKA Designs

In 2022, Ohlmeier et al. affirmed that in spite of the increasing number of publications reporting on the best surgical treatment in the management of PJI, there was no robust information regarding the type of infected prosthesis prior to any kind of exchange arthroplasty [12]. They studied the survivorship of non-hinged and hinged knee implants after one-stage exchange rTKA, the functional result after one-stage exchange procedure focusing on knee prostheses and the type of previous infected knee implant, and the potential influence of the type of femoral bone morphology measured by the inner femoral diameter on the rate of aseptic failures. Between January 2011 and December 2017, they analyzed 211 individuals with infected knee prostheses. Seventy-six percent (161 of 211 individuals) were accessible for final data analysis. These individuals were divided into four cohorts as per the performed implant revision: (1) bicondylar TKA to rotating-hinge implant, (2) rotating-hinge to rotating-hinge implant, (3) rotating-hinge to full hinge implant, and (4) full hinge to full hinge implant. The mean follow-up was 6 years, whereas a minimum follow-up of 3 years was required for inclusion. Survivorship and group analysis were carried out, and the functional result was evaluated utilizing postoperative OKSs at the latest follow-up (60-point scale with lower scores representing less pain and greater function). Moreover, in all individuals, femoral bone morphology was determined as per the Citak classification system [13]. At the final follow-up, the overall surgical revision rate was 23% with 9% suffering a PJI relapse. Cohort 1 consisted of 51, cohort 2 consisted of 67, cohort 3 consisted of 24, and cohort 4 consisted of 19 individuals. The lowest overall revision rate was encountered in cohort 2 (16%), compared with 28% in cohort 1, 29% in cohort 3, and 26% in cohort 4; however, no substantial differences were observed. The functional result (OKS) was clinically constant in all cohorts, with 32 points in cohort 1, 37 points in cohort 2, 33 points in cohort 3, and 35 points in cohort 4. Concerning the number of individuals with aseptic loosening as per bone morphology, 74% of all aseptic loosening cases appeared in femoral bone type C morphologies according to Citak (75% in cohort 1, 56% in cohort 2, 100% in cohort 3, and 100% in cohort 4). The results attained suggested a generally high overall revision rate (25%) with a good infection control rate (91%). Hinged implants reached more or less the same functional results and revision rates as nonhinged implants, when it comes to revision surgeries. The bone morphology, measured as per the Citak classification system, was confirmed as a risk factor for aseptic failures also in septic individuals [12].

8.4.8 PJI: Results of One-Stage Revision with Antibiotic-Impregnated Cancellous Bone Allograft

In 2022, Dersch et al. stated that debate existed concerning the optimal treatment of PJI, contemplating control of infection, functional outcomes, and quality of life. Difficulties in treatment come from the formation of biofilms within a few days following infection. Biofilms are tolerant to systemically given antibiotics, needing great concentrations for a lengthy period. Minimum biofilm eradication concentrations (MBEC) are only possible by the local employment of antibiotics. One proven strategy is the utilization of allograft bone as a carrier, bestowing a continuous liberation of antibiotics in very high concentrations after adequate impregnation [14]. In their study, Dersch et al. tried to determine the percentage of reinfection following a one-stage revision of infected hip or knee arthroplasties, utilizing antibiotic-impregnated allograft bone as the carrier and avoiding cement. They analyzed 70 individuals (34 male, 36 female) with a mean follow-up of 5.6 years and with a mean age of 68.2 years. Thirty-eight hips and 11 knees were implanted without any cement; and 21 knees were implanted with moderate cementing at the articular surface with stems always being uncemented. Within 2 years following surgery, 6 out of 70 individuals (8.6%) exhibited reinfection, and after more than 2 years, an additional 6 individuals exhibited late-onset infection. Within 2 years after surgery, 11 out of 70 individuals (15.7%) had an implant failure for any reason (including infection), and after more than 2 years, an additional 7 individuals had an implant failure. Using Kaplan-Meier analysis, the estimated survival for reinfection was 93.9% at 1 year, 89.9% at 2 years, and 81.5% at 5 years. The estimated survival for implant failure for any reason was 90.4% at 1 year, 80.9% at 2 years, and 71.1% at 5 years. One-stage revision with antibiotic-impregnated cancellous allograft bone bestows similar outcomes regarding infection control as with multiple stages [14].

8.5 High Revision Rates Following Repeat Septic Revision After Failed One-Stage Exchange for PJI in TKA

In 2022, Neufeld et al. affirmed that the result of repeat septic revision after a failed one-stage exchange for PJI in TKA endured undefined [15]. They reported the infection-free and all-cause revision-free survival of repeat septic revision after a failed one-stage exchange and try to discover whether the Musculoskeletal Infection Society (MSIS) [16] stage was associated with subsequent infection-related failure. Thirty-three repeat septic revisions (29 one-stage and 4 two-stage) were analyzed. The mean follow-up from repeat septic revision was 68.2 months. At the most recent follow-up, 17 repeat septic revisions (52%) had a subsequent infection-related failure, and the 5-year infection-free survival was 59%. Nineteen individuals experienced a subsequent all-cause revision (58%), and the 5-year all-cause revision-free survival was 47%. The most common indication for the first subsequent aseptic revision was loosening. The MSIS stage of the host status and limb status were not substantially related to subsequent infection-related failure. Repeat septic revision after a failed one-stage exchange TKA for PJI was associated with a high percentage of subsequent infection-related failure and all-cause revision [15].

8.6 Rate of Reinfection with Different and Difficult-to-Treat Bacteria After Failed One-Stage Septic Knee Exchange

In 2022, Akkaya et al. stated that reoperation after septic failure of a one-stage exchange for PJI of the knee is a greatly challenging technique with concerns over remaining osseous stock, soft tissues, and stability. The related changes in microbiology in cases of reinfection are still widely undefined [17]. A comprehensive analysis was carried out of all individuals treated between 2001 and 2017 who developed reinfection following a one-stage exchange for PJI of the knee. Requirements for inclusion were an unquestionable diagnosis of PJI according to the ICM (International Consensus Meeting) criteria [18] and a minimum follow-up of 3 years. Sixty-six individuals were recognized that met the inclusion criteria. Reinfection happened after a mean time interval of 27.7 months. Ten types of bacteria were encountered that were not present prior to the one-stage exchange. The causative microorganism endured alike in 22 individuals (33%) and additional pathogens were discovered in ten individuals (15%). However, 50% of the reinfections were due to (a) completely different pathogen(s). A substantial rise in the number of PJIs on the basis of high-virulent (23 versus 30) and difficult-to-treat bacteria (13 versus 24) was encountered [17].

8.7 Single-Stage rTKA Utilizing Intra-articular Antibiotic Infusion After Multiple Failed Surgeries for PJI

In 2022, Ji et al. analyzed the results of single-stage rTKA utilizing intra-articular antibiotic infusion in treating PJI [6]. They analyzed 78 PJI individuals (29 hips; 49 knees) who had experienced multiple previous surgical procedures. Their patients were treated with single-stage revision utilizing a supplementary intra-articular antibiotic infusion. Of these 78 individuals, 59 had experienced more than two previous failed debridement and implant retentions, 12 individuals had a failed arthroplasty resection, three hips had previously experienced failed two-stage revision, and four had a failed one-stage revision prior to their single-stage revision. Previous failure was defined as infection recurrence needing surgical intervention. Additionally, in intravenous pathogen-sensitive drugs, an intra-articular infusion of vancomycin, imipenem, or voriconazole was carried out postoperatively. The antibiotic solution was soaked into the joint for 24 h for a mean of 16 days and then extracted prior to next injection. Sixty-eight individuals (87.1%) were free of infection at a mean follow-up time of 85 months. The 7-year infection-free survival was 87.6%. No substantial difference in infection-free survival was seen between hip and knee PJIs (91.5% (95% versus 84.7%). The mean postoperative Harris Hip Score was 76.1 points and Hospital for Special Surgery (HSS) score was 78.2 at the most recent evaluation. Polymicrobial and fungal infections accounted for 14.1% and 9% of all cases, respectively. Single-stage revision with intra-articular antibiotic infusion can render elevated antibiotic concentration in synovial fluid, therefore overcoming diminished vascular supply and biofilm formation. This supplementary route of administration might be a viable alternative in managing PJI after multiple failed prior surgical procedures for reinfection [6].

8.8 Varus-Valgus Constrained Implant Following One-Stage rTKA for PJI

In 2023, Ji et al. assessed the mid-run survival of varus-valgus constrained (VVC) implants utilized in one-stage rTKA for PJI [3]. They analyzed 132 individuals with chronic PJI who experienced one-stage revision utilizing a VVC implant. The average follow-up was 51.6 months. Five-year survival analysis was carried out to set recurrent infection and mechanical failure as the end point. HSS as functional results was assessed preoperatively and at the latest follow-up. A total of 12 individuals (9.1%) experienced retreatment for reinfection (nine individuals) and mechanical failure (three individuals). The overall 5-year revision-free survival was 82.7%, the infection-free survival was 91.1%, and the mechanical failure-free survival was 98.3%. The preoperative HSS knee score improved from 35.6 points before surgery to 76.8 points at the latest follow-up. Adverse events were recognized in 20 individuals (15.2%) which included aseptic osteolysis in four cases, acceptable flexion instability in three cases, arthrofibrosis in two individuals, hematomas in two cases, calf intermuscular venous thrombosis in six individuals, and femoral stem tip pain in three cases. Improved functional result and good mid-run survival were shown at an average follow-up of 51.6 months [3].

8.9 Comparison of Reinfection Rates and Other Clinical Outcomes Between One-Stage and the Two-Stage rTKA

In a systematic review and meta-analysis published in 2016 by Kunutsor et al., they stated that PJI was a severe adverse event of TKA. Two-stage revision was the most commonly utilized surgical technique and contemplated as the most efficacious for managing PJI of the knee. The one-stage revision approach was an emerging alternative option; however, its performance in comparison to the two-stage approach was unclear [19]. They studied if there was a difference in reinfection percentages and other clinical results when comparing the one-stage to the two-stage revision approach. Their first goal was to compare reinfection (new and recurrent infections) percentages for one- and two-stage revision surgery for PJI of the knee. Their second goal was to compare between the two revision approaches, clinical results as measured by postoperative KS knee score, KS function score, HSS knee score, WOMAC (Western Ontario and McMaster Universities Osteoarthritis Index) score, and ROM. The rate of reinfection was 7.6% in one-stage studies. The corresponding reinfection rate for two-stage revision was 8.8%. Postoperative clinical results of knee scores and ROM were similar for both revision approaches. This study suggested the one-stage revision approach might be as efficacious as the two-stage revision approach in managing infected knee prostheses in generally unselected individuals [19].

8.10 Conclusions

PJI of the knee represents a severe complication after 1.5–2% of pTKAs. rTKA is challenging to carry out in individuals with PJI because of the difficulty of eliminating the infection and possibility for osseous and ligamentous deficits. Two-stage revision has traditionally been contemplated the gold standard of treatment for proven infection, but growing proof is coming out in support of one-stage exchange for selected individuals. One-stage exchange is indicated when there is no sign of systemic sepsis and in cases where a microorganism has been isolated. It involves removal of the old prosthesis, debridement of all infected tissue, a copious washout and redraping, and finally, reimplantation of a new prosthesis. Contraindications to the procedure are systemic sepsis, large osseous or soft tissue loss, extensor mechanism failure, or if primary wound closure is improbable to be attainable.

In a recent systematic review, a reinfection rate of 12.2% after an average follow-up of 57.6 months was found. The most common causative pathogens were gram-positive bacteria (71.1%), gram-negative bacteria (7.1%), and polymicrobial infections (8%). The infection-free survival following management for repeating infection was 92.1%. The causative pathogens at reinfections differed substantially from the primary infection (gram-positive 44.4%, gram-negative 11.1%). Individuals who experienced a one-stage rTKA for PJI exhibited a reinfection percentage inferior or comparable to other surgical treatments as two-stage or DAIR.

References

1. Ciccullo C, Neri T, Farinelli L, Gigante A, Philippot R, Farizon F, et al. Antibiotic prophylaxis in one-stage revision of septic total knee arthroplasty: a scoping review. Antibiotics (Basel). 2023;12(3):606. https://doi.org/10.3390/antibiotics12030606.
2. Bosco F, Cacciola G, Giustra F, Risitano S, Capella M, Vezza D, et al. Characterizing recurrent infections after one-stage revision for periprosthetic joint infection of the knee: a systematic review of the literature. Eur J Orthop Surg Traumatol. 2023;33(7):2703–15. https://doi.org/10.1007/s00590-023-03480-7.
3. Ji B, Li G, Zhang X, Wang Y, Mu W, Cao L. Midterm survival of a varus-valgus constrained implant following one-stage revision for periprosthetic joint infection: a single-center study. J Knee Surg. 2023;36(3):284–91. https://doi.org/10.1055/s-0041-1731739.

4. Razii N, Clutton JM, Kakar R, Morgan-Jones R. Single-stage revision for the infected total knee arthroplasty: the Cardiff experience. Bone Jt Open. 2021;2(5):305–13. https://doi.org/10.1302/2633-1462.25.BJO-2020-0185.R1.
5. Wignadasan W, Ibrahim M, Haddad FS. One- or two-stage reimplantation for infected total knee prosthesis? Orthop Traumatol Surg Res. 2023;109(1S):103453. https://doi.org/10.1016/j.otsr.2022.103453.
6. Ji B, Li G, Zhang X, Xu B, Wang Y, Chen Y, et al. Effective single-stage revision using intra-articular antibiotic infusion after multiple failed surgery for periprosthetic joint infection: a mean seven years' follow-up. Bone Joint J. 2022;104-B(7):867–74. https://doi.org/10.1302/0301-620X.104B7.BJJ-2021-1704.R1.
7. Thakrar RR, Horriat S, Kayani B, Haddad FS. Indications for a single-stage exchange arthroplasty for chronic prosthetic joint infection: a systematic review. Bone Joint J. 2019;101-B(1_Supple_A):19–24. https://doi.org/10.1302/0301-620X.101B1.BJJ-2018-0374.R1.
8. Li F, Qiao Y, Zhang H, Cao G, Zhou S. Comparable clinical outcomes of culture-negative and culture-positive periprosthetic joint infections: a systematic review and meta-analysis. J Orthop Surg Res. 2023;18(1):210. https://doi.org/10.1186/s13018-023-03692-x.
9. Rossmann M, Minde T, Citak M, Gehrke T, Sandiford NA, Klatte TO, et al. High rate of reinfection with new bacteria following one-stage exchange for enterococcal periprosthetic infection of the knee: a single-center study. J Arthroplasty. 2021;36(2):711–6. https://doi.org/10.1016/j.arth.2020.08.015.
10. Ohlmeier M, Alrustom F, Citak M, Salber J, Gehrke T, Frings J. What is the mid-term survivorship of infected rotating-hinge implants treated with one-stage-exchange? Clin Orthop Relat Res. 2021;479(12):2714–22. https://doi.org/10.1097/CORR.0000000000001868.
11. Pellegrini A, Meani E, Macchi V, Legnani C. One-stage revision surgery provides infection eradication and satisfying outcomes for infected knee arthroplasty in selected patients. Expert Rev Anti Infect Ther. 2021;19(7):945–8. https://doi.org/10.1080/14787210.2021.1851597.
12. Ohlmeier M, Alrustom F, Citak M, Rolvien T, Gehrke T, Frings J. The clinical outcome of different total knee arthroplasty designs in one-stage revision for periprosthetic infection. J Arthroplasty. 2022;37(2):359–66. https://doi.org/10.1016/j.arth.2021.10.002.
13. Citak M, Levent A, Suero EM, Rademacher K, Busch S-M, Gehrke T. A novel radiological classification system of the distal femur. Arch Orthop Trauma Surg. 2022;142(2):315–22. https://doi.org/10.1007/s00402-021-03828-w.
14. Dersch G, Winkler H. Periprosthetic joint infection (PJI)-results of one-stage revision with antibiotic-impregnated cancellous allograft bone—a retrospective cohort study. Antibiotics (Basel). 2022;11(3):310. https://doi.org/10.3390/antibiotics11030310.
15. Neufeld ME, Liechti EF, Soto F, Linke P, Busch SM, Gehrke T, et al. High revision rates following repeat septic revision after failed one-stage exchange for periprosthetic joint infection in total knee arthroplasty. Bone Joint J. 2022;104-B(3):386–93. https://doi.org/10.1302/0301-620X.104B3.BJJ-2021-0481.R2.
16. Parvizi J, Tan TL, Goswami K, Higuera C, Della Valle C, Chen AF, et al. The 2018 definition of periprosthetic hip and knee infection: an evidence-based and validated criteria. J Arthroplasty. 2018;33(5):1309–1314.e2. https://doi.org/10.1016/j.arth.2018.02.078.
17. Akkaya M, Vles G, Bakhtiari IG, Sandiford A, Salber J, Gehrke T, et al. What is the rate of reinfection with different and difficult-to-treat bacteria after failed one-stage septic knee exchange? Int Orthop. 2022;46(4):687–95. https://doi.org/10.1007/s00264-021-05291-z.
18. Parvizi J, Gehrke T, Chen AF. Proceedings of the international consensus on periprosthetic joint infection. Bone Joint J. 2013;95-B(11):1450–2. https://doi.org/10.1302/0301-620X.95B11.33135.
19. Kunutsor SK, Whitehouse MR, Lenguerrand E, Blom AW, Beswick AD, INFORM Team. Re-infection outcomes following one- and two-stage surgical revision of infected knee prosthesis: a systematic review and meta-analysis. PLoS One. 2016;11(3):e0151537. https://doi.org/10.1371/journal.pone.0151537.

Two-Stage Revision Total Knee Arthroplasty for Periprosthetic Joint Infection

9

E. Carlos Rodríguez-Merchán, Carlos A. Encinas-Ullán, Juan S. Ruiz-Pérez, and Primitivo Gómez-Cardero

9.1 Introduction

Periprosthetic joint infection (PJI) following total knee arthroplasty (TKA) is one of the most disastrous and expensive adverse events that carries substantial patient wellness as well as economic burdens. The way to effectively diagnosing and managing PJI is challenging, as there is still no gold standard approach to achieve the diagnosis as early as wanted. There are also debates with respect to the best strategy to treat PJI cases [1]. In this chapter, recent advances in managing PJI following TKA by means of the two-stage revision approach are reviewed.

9.2 The Importance of ESR, CRP, WBC Count, and the Strip Test

9.2.1 The Importance of ESR and CRP Before Second-Stage Reimplantation Knee Revision Surgery

According to Klemt et al., although two-stage revision surgery is considered as the most efficacious treatment for managing chronic PJI, there is no current accord on the predictors of optimal timing to second-stage reimplantation [2]. They compared clinical results between individuals with elevated erythrocyte sedimentation rate (ESR) and C-reactive protein (CRP) before second-stage reimplantation and those with normalized ESR and CRP before second-stage reimplantation. They analyzed 198 individuals treated with two-stage revision TKA (rTKA) for chronic PJI. Groups included individuals with normal level of serum ESR and CRP ($N = 96$) and

---

E. C. Rodríguez-Merchán (✉) · C. A. Encinas-Ullán · J. S. Ruiz-Pérez · P. Gómez-Cardero
Department of Orthopedic Surgery, La Paz University Hospital, Madrid, Spain

© The Author(s), under exclusive license to Springer Nature Switzerland AG 2024
E. C. Rodríguez-Merchán (ed.), *Advances in Revision Total Knee Arthroplasty*,
https://doi.org/10.1007/978-3-031-60445-4_9

elevated level of serum ESR and CRP before second-stage reimplantation ($N = 102$). Results including reinfection percentages and readmission percentages were compared between both groups. At a mean follow-up of 4.4 years, the elevated ESR and CRP group showed substantially higher reinfection percentages compared with individuals with normalized ESR and CRP before second-stage reimplantation (33.3% versus 14.5%). Individuals with both elevated ESR and CRP showed substantially higher reinfection percentages, when compared with individuals with elevated ESR and normalized CRP (33.3% versus 27.6%) as well as normalized ESR and elevated CRP (33.3% versus 26.3%). Klemt et al. demonstrated that high serum ESR and CRP levels before reimplantation in two-stage knee rTKA for chronic PJI were associated with increased reinfection percentage after surgery. Elevation of both ESR and CRP were associated with a higher risk of reinfection compared with elevation of either ESR or CRP, denoting the possible benefits of normalizing ESR and CRP before reimplantation in management of chronic PJI [2].

9.2.2 Synovial WBC Count and Polymorphonuclear Differential Thresholds

In a study published in 2022 by Pannu et al., synovial white blood cell (WBC) count showed very high specificity to confirm successful reimplantation. Both WBC count and polymorphonuclear differential (PMN%) can significantly determine reimplantation survival. They analyzed 88 two-stage hip/knee arthroplasties. Synovial PMN% exhibited superior accuracy than WBC count in determining result of reimplantation. The optimal PMN% threshold (62%) showed sensitivity of 57% and specificity of 77%. The estimated WBC count threshold (2733/μL) demonstrated poor sensitivity (21%) but high specificity (95%). There was a substantial difference in failure-free survival (24 months) between the cases with WBC count higher versus lower than 2733/μL. This was also true for PMN% at 5 months postoperatively [3].

9.2.3 CRP and WBC Count

According to Benda et al., in septic two-stage revision arthroplasty, the timing of reimplantation is essential for therapeutic success. Recent studies had demonstrated that singular values of CRP and WBC count display weak diagnostic value in indicating whether PJI is controlled or not during two-stage rTKA. Thus, besides the values of CRP and WBC, the course of CRP and WBC counts were compared between cohorts with and without later reinfection in 95 individuals with two-stage rTKA of infected TKAs. Of these individuals, 16 had a reinfection (16.84%). CRP values diminished substantially after the first stage of two-stage rTKA in both the reinfection and no-reinfection cohorts. WBC count values diminished substantially in the no-reinfection cohort. Reduction in WBC count was not substantial in the reinfection cohort. No substantial difference could be encountered in either the CRP values or the WBC counts at the first stage of two-stage revision, the second stage of two-stage revision, or their difference between stages when comparing cohorts with and without reinfection. The courses of CRP over 14 days after the first stage of both cohorts were similar. CRP and WBC count as well as their course over 14 days postoperatively were not appropriate for defining whether a PJI of the knee is under control or not [4].

9.2.4 The Strip Test Renders a Helpful Intraoperative Diagnostic During Second-Stage Revision for PJI

In 2022, Logoluso et al. assessed the dependability of intraoperative evaluation of leukocyte esterase (LE) in synovial fluid samples from individuals experiencing reimplantation following implant removal and spacer insertion for PJI. Their hypothesis was that a positive intraoperative LE test would be a better predictor of persistent infection than either serum CRP or ESR or the combination of serum CRP and ESR. They analyzed 76 individuals who underwent two-stage exchange for PJI. Synovial fluid was collected for LE measurement during surgery before arthrotomy in 79 procedures. Sensitivity, specificity, positive predictive value, and negative predictive value of the LE assay were 82%, 99%, 90%, and 97%, respectively. The best thresholds for the CRP and the ESR assay were 8.25 mg/L (82% sensitivity, 84% specificity) and 45 mm/h (55% sensitivity, 87% specificity), respectively. The LE strip test proved a dependable method to diagnose persistence of infection and outperformed the serum CRP and ESR assays. The strip test rendered a helpful intraoperative diagnostic during second-stage revision for PJI [5].

9.3 Static Versus Dynamic Spacers

In 2022, Craig et al. reported that the use of antibiotic-eluting polymethylmethacrylate (PMMA) articular spacers in two-stage rTKA for PJI accomplishes a high rate of infection eradication (>80%). Dynamic spacers might give a diversity of benefits compared to static spacers, with a similar percentage of infection eradication [6].

9.3.1 All-Cement Articulating Spacers and Sterilized Replanted Metal-Polyethylene Articulating Spacers

In 2022, Fei et al. compared the results of all-cement articulating spacers and sterilized replanted metal-polyethylene articulating spacers for PJI following TKA. Forty-seven individuals were categorized as receiving an all-cement articulating spacer or a sterilized replanted metal-polyethylene articulating spacer in exclusion. Forty-seven spacers were recognized: all-cement spacer was used in 23 individuals and sterilized replanted spacer in 24. Individuals in the all-cement spacer cohort had shorter operation time (155.87 versus 189.79 min) and less blood loss (845.22 versus 1114.50 mL) in exclusion. Individuals in the sterilized replanted spacer cohort had superior interval range of motion (range of motion, ROM; 61° versus 31.75°) and postoperative ROM (85° versus 77.37°) as compared to all-cement spacers, but there was no difference in infection control between two cohorts. The two types of spacers had no difference in the reinfection percentage, indicating that both articulating spacers are safe and efficacious for two-stage rTKA. Taking into account ROM of the knee joint, bone loss, and cost, sterilized replanted metal-polyethylene spacers were preferred in the management of PJI [7].

9.4 Predictors of Failure

In 2022, Russo et al. affirmed that in spite of the standardization of two-stage rTKA protocols, a high percentage of failures still occur. Recognizing the predictors of failure is needed to determine adequate treatment and counsel for individuals with a PJI of the knee. Russo et al. aimed to recognize risk factors forecasting the failure, to describe implant survival, and to report the mid-run clinical results of individuals experiencing two-stage rTKA for PJI. Data of individuals who experienced two-stage knee revision from 2012 to 2016 were analyzed, and 108 individuals were included. The mean age was 66.6 years. The mean follow-up was 52.9 months. Difficult-to-treat infections, the number of prior surgeries, and the level of tibial bone defect substantially forecasted the failure of two-stage rTKA. Survivorship of implants was substantially lower for individuals presenting these risk factors [8].

9.4.1 Predictors of Reinfection

In 2022, Hartman et al. examined the relationship between patient risk factors, comorbidities, and the pathogen on reinfection percentages after two-stage rTKA. They assessed 158 individuals treated for PJI from 2008 to 2019. Only individuals who had completed a two-stage exchange were included. Thirty-one individuals experienced a reinfection (19.6%). There was a statistically significant association between infection with methicillin-sensitive *Staphylococcus aureus* (MSSA) and reinfection. Individuals with a reinfection also had a significantly greater median serum CRP level (12.65 g/dL) at the time of diagnosis compared to individuals without a reinfection (5 g/dL). Median ESR (56 in no reinfection and 69 in reinfection) and time to reimplantation (101 days in no reinfection and 141 days in reinfection) showed a tendency toward an association with reinfection but were not statistically significant. As the number of TKAs continues to increase, PJIs are rising proportionately and represent a substantial revision burden. Elevated CRP levels and MSSA infection were strongly associated with failure of a two-stage rTKA. Besides, there were strong tendencies toward an association between elevated ESR, longer time to reimplantation, and reinfection [9].

9.4.2 Rifampicin Resistance and Risk Factors Associated with Significantly Lower Recovery Rates

In 2022, Krizsan et al. stated that rifampicin plays a key role in the management of PJIs; however, the emergence of rifampicin resistance is associated with less favorable clinical results. That was why they investigated the influence of rifampicin resistance and other patient-related factors on recovery percentages among individuals with PJI experiencing two-stage rTKA. They found that rifampicin resistance was associated with lower recovery percentages among individuals experiencing two-stage rTKA due to PJI. Higher age and type 2 diabetes mellitus had negative influence on clinical result [10].

9.5 Results

9.5.1 Long-Run Reinfection, Adverse Event, and Mortality

In 2022, Kildow et al. analyzed the long-run reinfection, adverse event, and mortality following two-stage rTKA. They reviewed 178 individuals who experienced two-stage rTKA for chronic PJI. Overall rate of infection eradication was 85.41%, with a mortality rate of 30.33%. Individuals with minimum 5-year follow-up ($N = 118$, average 8.32 years) had an infection eradication rate of 88.98%, with a mortality rate of 33.05% [11].

9.5.2 Factors that Affect Range of Motion

In 2022, Kim et al. evaluated factors that affect ROM following 98 two-stage rTKAs as a treatment for chronic PJI of the knee. ROM after the first-stage surgery, whether a reoperation was carried out prior to the second-stage surgery, the interval between the first-stage surgery and the second-stage surgery, and body mass index (BMI) were encountered to be factors that were associated with ROM after two-stage rTKA [12].

9.5.3 The Impact of Diabetes Mellitus

In 2022, Lin et al. tried to clarify the importance of preoperative glycated hemoglobin (HbA1c) levels before each stage of revision arthroplasty and analyzed the risk factors for reinfection. Five hundred eighty-eight individuals that suffered from first-time PJI were reviewed. The mean follow-up time was 13.8 years. Patients who experienced two-stage rTKA with diabetes mellitus at presentation were included. The end point of the study was reinfection of the rTKA. Eighty-eight individuals were recognized and grouped by HbA1c level prior to the first stage surgery: Cohorts 1 and 2 had HbA1c levels <7% and ≥7%, respectively. Reinfection was recognized in 4.55% (2/44) and 18.18% (8/44) of the individuals in cohorts 1 and 2, respectively. Survivorship analysis revealed correction of the HbA1c prior to the final stage of rTKA as an independent factor. The recognized risks for reinfection were HbA1c levels ≥7% prior to final-stage surgery, ≥3 stages of revision arthroplasty, and extended-spectrum beta-lactamase (ESBL)-producing *Escherichia coli* PJI. The HbA1c level prior the final stage of revision arthroplasty could influence staged rTKA results [13].

9.5.4 Clinical Efficacy

In 2022, Qiao et al. explored the clinical influence of two-stage revision surgery for the treatment of PJI after TKA. The clinical data of 27 individuals (3 males and 24 females; mean age, 66.7 years; 27 knees) with PJI treated with two-stage revision surgery were analyzed retrospectively. All 27 patients were followed up (range, 13–112 months). The ESR (14.5 mm/h) and CRP (0.6 mg/dL) of the individuals at the last follow-up were substantially lower than those at admission; the difference was statistically significant. The postoperative visual analogue scale (VAS) score (1.1), Hospital for Special Surgery (HSS) score (82.3), and knee ROM (108°) were substantially improved compared with those before the surgery; the difference was statistically significant. Of the 27 patients, 26 were cured of the infection, whereas one case had an infection recurrence; the infection control rate was 96.3%. Two-stage revision surgery can effectively alleviate pain, control infection, and retain good joint function in the management of PJI after TKA [14]. Figures 9.1, 9.2, and 9.3 show three cases of septic loosening of TKA treated by two-stage revision arthroplasty. Figure 9.3 shows a dislocation of the articulated spacer as a complication of this type of surgery.

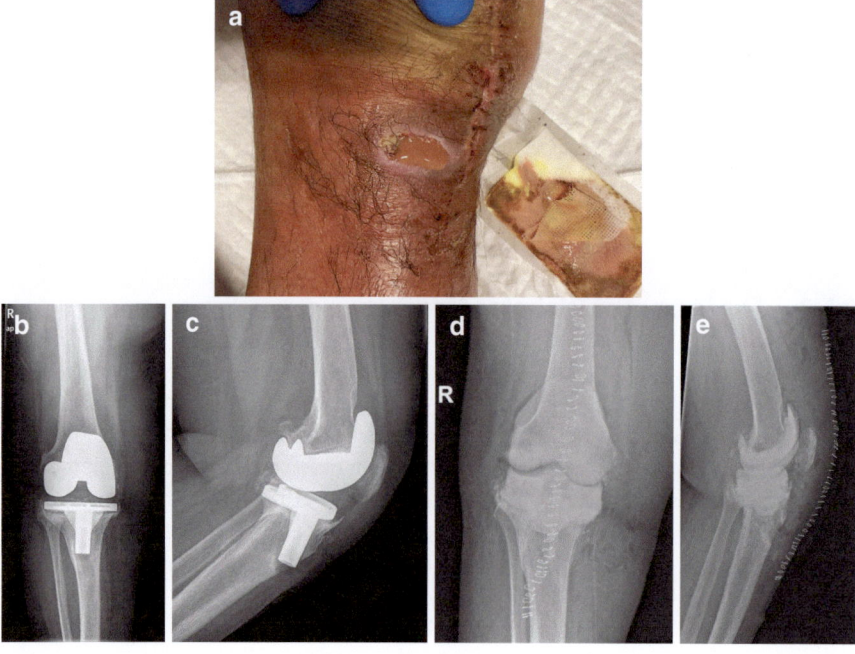

Fig. 9.1 (**a–e**) Septic loosening of total knee arthroplasty (TKA): chronic fistula (**a**); anteroposterior (AP) (**b**) and lateral (**c**) radiographs show clear signs of loosening; in the first revision arthroplasty time, an articulated spacer was placed, as shown in the AP (**d**) and lateral (**e**) radiographic images after the first stage of two-stage revision arthroplasty

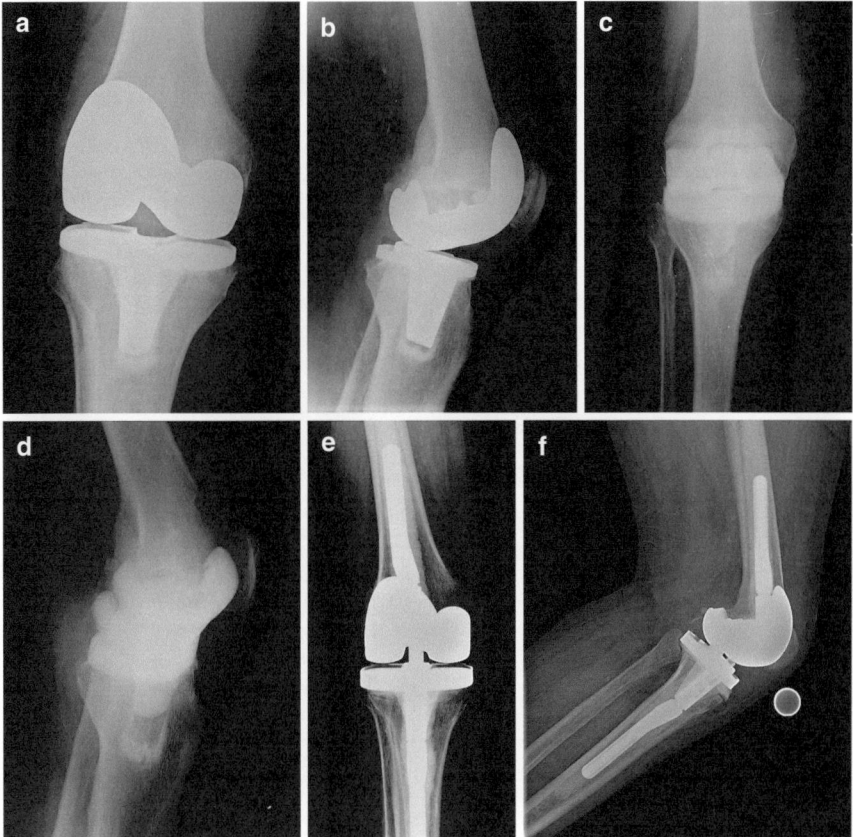

Fig. 9.2 (**a–f**) Anteroposterior (AP) (**a**) and lateral (**b**) radiographic images of septic loosening due to *Staphylococcus pyogenes*; in the first-stage revision arthroplasty, an articulated spacer was implanted, as shown in the AP (**c**) and lateral (**d**) radiographic images after such intervention; in the second-stage revision arthroplasty, a CCK (constrained condylar knee) was implanted, as shown in the AP (**e**) and lateral (**f**) radiographic images after such intervention

9.5.5 Relationship Between Preresection Nutrition and Success After First-Stage Resection in Planned Two-Stage Exchange for PJI

According to Green et al., nutritionally compromised individuals, with preoperative serum albumin (SAB) < 3.5 g/dL, are at higher risk for PJI in TKA. The relationship between nutritional and PJI treatment success is unknown. Therefore, in 99 knees, they examined the relationship between preresection nutrition and success after first-stage resection in planned two-stage exchange for PJI. Failure was defined as persistent infection or repeat surgery for infection after resection. Among individuals with preoperative SAB > 3.5 g/dL, the failure rate was 32% versus a 48% failure

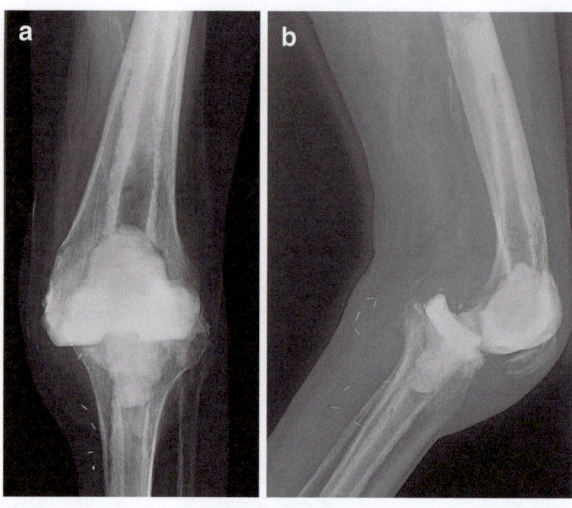

Fig. 9.3 (**a**, **b**) Dislocation of the articulated spacer implanted in the first-stage revision arthroplasty of an infected total knee arthroplasty (TKA): anteroposterior radiograph (**a**); lateral view (**b**)

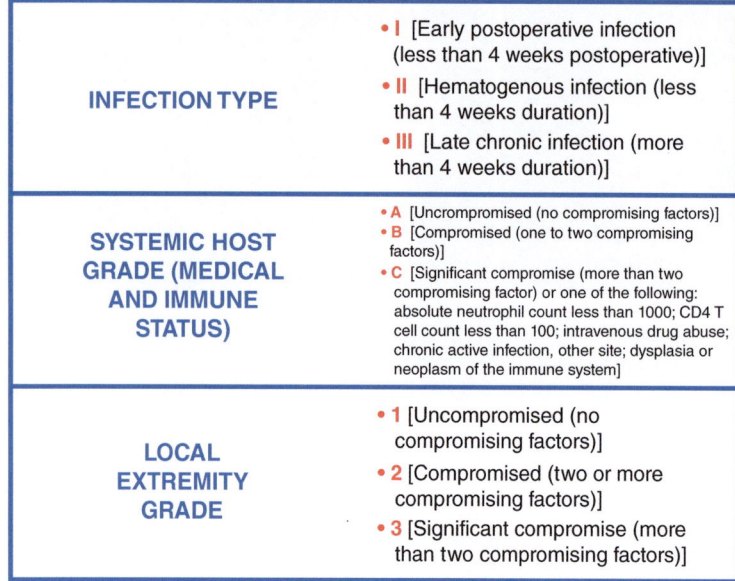

Fig. 9.4 Staging system for periprosthetic joint infection (PJI)

rate when SAB < 3.5 g/dL. Multivariable regression results indicated that preoperative low SAB (< 3.5 g/dL) and Musculoskeletal Infection Society (MSIS) host type-C [15] (Figs. 9.4 and 9.5) were independent risk factors for failure following first-stage resection in planned two-stage rTKA for PJI [16].

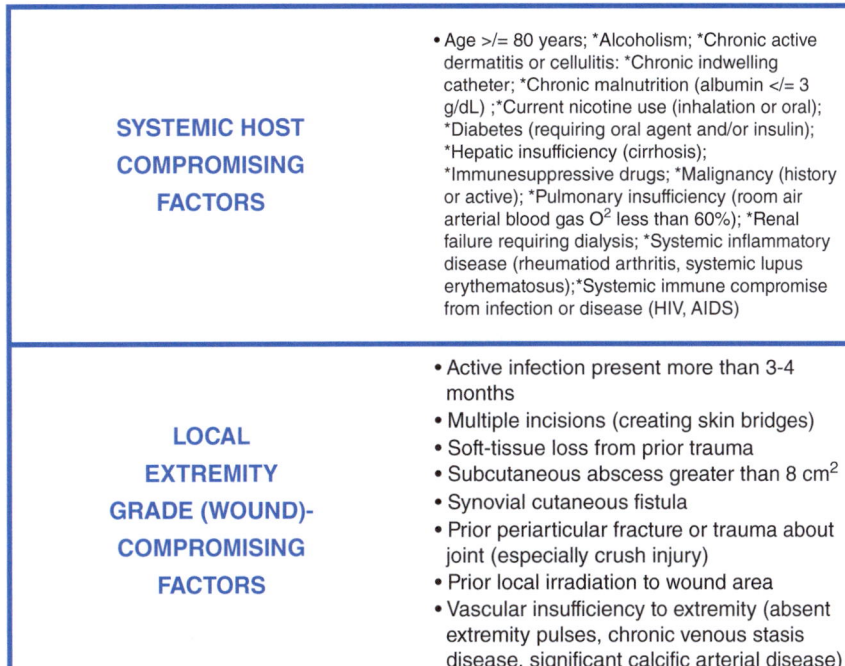

Fig. 9.5 Compromising factors for periprosthetic joint infection (PJI)

9.6 Megaprosthetic Distal Femoral Reconstruction Compared to Hinged TKA

In a study with level 4 of evidence published in 2022, Theil et al. analyzed the survival of distal femoral reconstruction (DFR) compared to hinged TKA in 97 individuals who experienced two-stage revision due to chronic knee PJI. Among these, 41 were DFR. The diagnosis of PJI was determined utilizing the MSIS criteria. The median follow-up period was 59 months. Overall, 24% of individuals needed revision surgery for infection. The infection-free survival of rotating hinge revision TKA was 93% at 5 years compared to 50% for DFR. The risk factors for reinfection were DFR reconstruction, length of megaprosthesis, and higher BMI. Ten percent of individuals experiencing DFR underwent amputation to manage recurrent infection. Megaprosthetic DFR as part of a two-stage exchange for PJI is a salvage treatment that has an elevated risk for reinfection compared to non-megaprosthetic TKA [17].

9.7 Structural Fresh Frozen Allogenous Bone Grafts in Managing Patients in Knee PJI with Large Bone Defects

According to Chuang et al., the revision surgeries for knee PJI might become more challenging when it is associated with large bone defects. They investigated the result of structural fresh frozen allogenous bone grafts in managing individuals in knee PJI with large bone defects. Twelve individuals with structural allogenous bone graft reconstructions were identified as the study cohort. Twenty-four individuals without structural allograft reconstructions matched with the study cohort by age, gender, and Charlson Comorbidity Index [18] were enrolled as the control cohort. The functional result of the study cohort was assessed with the Knee Society Score (KSS). Treatment success was evaluated according to the Delphi-based consensus definition. The infection relapse percentage and implant survivorship were compared between cohorts. Revision knees with structural allograft showed excellent improvement in the KSS (33.1–75.4). There was no substantial difference between infection relapse-free survival percentage and prosthesis survival percentage in the two cohorts. The 8-year prosthesis survival percentage was 90.9% in the study cohort and 91% in the control cohort. The 8-year infection relapse-free survival percentage was 80 and 83.3% in the study cohort and control cohort, respectively. The structural fresh frozen allogenous bone graft rendered an efficacious way for bone defect reconstruction in knee PJI with an accountable survival percentage. Meanwhile, utilizing structural allografts did not increase the relapse percentage of infection [19].

9.8 Repeat Two-Stage Revision

According to Christiner et al. (2022), two-stage rTKA is the gold standard for treatment and eradication of knee PJI, but the literature is limited on the results of repeat two-stage TKA after PJI recurrence. In their study, they presented the results of repeat two-stage revision TKA and investigated potential factors contributing to success or failure. Twenty cases experienced repeat two-stage rTKA. Patient results and factors contributing to treatment success or failure were studied. PJI was diagnosed according to MSIS criteria. Of the 20 cases, 14 were classified as failed treatment (70%) because of a failure to eradicate infection, further surgical intervention, or death. In this group, there were no statistically significant differences between the cohorts regarding factors contributing to management success or failure. In the success cohort, patient-reported functional results were variable. This study showed that individuals experiencing a repeat two-stage TKA have very poor results. This study did not identify any factors that forecast failure. Individuals need to be counseled regarding poor results with repeat two-stage TKA, and other treatment alternatives such as early amputation or lifelong suppression should be considered [20].

In 2023, Steinicke et al. affirmed that management of recurrent infection after a two-stage exchange remained debated, and the result of a repeat two-stage procedure was unclear. They investigated the success percentages of repeat two-stage exchange arthroplasty and analyzed potential risk factors for failure. They identified 55 individuals (23 hips, 32 knees) who were treated with repeat resection arthroplasty and planned delayed reimplantation for recurrent PJI after a previous two-stage revision. The minimum follow-up was 12 months. Seventy-eight percent experienced reimplantation after a repeat implant removal. Of those who completed the second-stage surgery, 37% experienced additional revision for infection, and 14% experienced amputation. The reinfection-free implant survivorship amounted to 77% after 1 year and 38% after 5 years. Individuals with a higher comorbidity score were less likely to experience second-stage reimplantation (median 5 versus 3). Moreover, obese individuals and diabetics had a higher risk for further infection. Most frequently, cultures yielded polymicrobial growth at the repeat two-stage exchange (27%) and at re-reinfection (32%). Pathogen persistence was found in 21% of re-reinfected individuals. The success percentages after repeat two-stage exchange arthroplasty were low [21].

9.9 One-Stage Versus Two-Stage Septic Revision of TKA

According to Wignadasan et al., a PJI is possibly the most substantial potential adverse event of TKA and is associated with significant morbidity and socioeconomic burden. It is a devastating adverse event for both the individual and the surgeon alike. A two-stage revision procedure for infected TKA has been the standard for surgical management; however, there is growing interest in single-stage revision surgery due to fewer procedures, diminished inpatient hospital stay, and diminished costs to healthcare systems. A one-stage exchange is indicated when there is no sign of systemic sepsis and in cases where a pathogen has been isolated. It entails removal of the old implant, debridement of all infected tissue, an abundant washout and redraping, and finally, re-implantation of a new prosthesis. The two-stage approach entails the employment of an antibiotic spacer prior to the second stage is performed. Individuals with a PJI should be managed by a multidisciplinary team. Wignadasan et al. recommended these individuals are managed in specialist arthroplasty centers by high volume rTKA specialists [22].

9.9.1 Mortality and Re-revision Following Single-Stage and Two-Stage Revision Surgery

In 2022, Lenguerrand et al. compared the risks of re-revision and mortality between two-stage revision surgery and single-stage revision surgery among individuals with infected primary TKA. Individuals with a PJI of their primary TKA (pTKA), initially revised with a single-stage or a two-stage procedure in England and Wales between 2003 and 2014, were identified from the National Joint Registry. A total of 489 pTKAs were revised with single-stage procedure (1390 person-years) and 2377 with two-stage procedure (8349 person-years). The adjusted incidence percentages of all-cause re-revision and for infection were comparable between these strategies. Individuals initially managed with single-stage revision received fewer revision procedures overall than after two-stage revision (1.2 versus 2.2). Mortality was lower for single-stage revision between 6 and 18 months postoperative and comparable at other timepoints. The risk of re-revision was similar between single- and two-stage revision for infected primary TKA. Single-stage cohort needed fewer revisions overall, with lower or comparable mortality at specific postoperative periods. The single-stage revision was a safe and efficacious approach to manage infected TKAs. There is potential for increased employment to diminish the burden of knee PJI for individuals and for the healthcare system [23].

9.9.2 Is Two-Stage Septic Revision Worth the Money?

In 2023, Okafor et al. stated that two-stage rTKA remains the gold standard for the treatment of PJI of the knee, but several studies have shown that one-stage exchange is as efficacious as two-stage exchange. This study aimed to support decision-making via an economic assessment of one-stage compared to two-stage exchange for TKA septic revision in individuals who did not have compelling indication PJI (i.e., methicillin-resistant *Staphylococcus aureus* (MRSA), multiorganism, systemic sepsis, comorbidities, culture negative, resistant organism, and immunocompromised) to experience a two-stage exchange. A cost-utility analysis was carried out utilizing a Markov cohort model. The adoption of one-stage septic knee revision is the optimal choice for individuals who have a PJI and who do not have a compelling need for a two-stage rTKA. One-stage exchange for PJI should be recommended in individuals who meet the eligibility criteria [24].

9.10 Conclusions

Difficult-to-treat infections, the number of prior surgeries, and the level of tibial bone defect substantially forecast the failure of two-stage rTKA. Survivorship of implants is substantially lower for individuals presenting these risk factors. A study demonstrated that high serum ESR and CRP levels before reimplantation in two-stage knee rTKA for chronic PJI were associated with increased reinfection percentage after surgery. Elevation of both ESR and CRP were associated with a higher risk of reinfection compared with elevation of either ESR or CRP. The LE strip test proves a dependable method to diagnose persistence of infection and outperformed the serum CRP and ESR assays. The strip test renders a helpful intraoperative diagnostic during second-stage revision for PJI. The use of antibiotic-eluting PMMA articular spacers in two-stage rTKA for PJI accomplishes a high rate of infection eradication (>80%). Elevated CRP levels and MSSA infection are strongly associated with failure of a two-stage rTKA. Besides, there are strong tendencies toward an association between elevated ESR, longer time to reimplantation, and reinfection. The recognized risks for reinfection are HbA1c levels ≥7% prior to final-stage surgery, ≥3 stages of revision arthroplasty, and extended-spectrum beta-lactamase (ESBL)-producing *Escherichia coli* PJI. The HbA1c level prior the final stage of revision arthroplasty could influence staged rTKA results. Preoperative low SAB (<3.5 g/dL) and MSIS host type-C are independent risk factors for failure following first-stage resection in planned two-stage rTKA for PJI.

References

1. Alrayes MM, Sukeik M. Two-stage revision in periprosthetic knee joint infections. World J Orthop. 2023;14(3):113–22. https://doi.org/10.5312/wjo.v14.i3.113.
2. Klemt C, Padmanabha A, Esposito JG, Laurencin S, Smith EJ, Kwon YM. Elevated ESR and CRP prior to second-stage reimplantation knee revision surgery for periprosthetic joint infection are associated with increased reinfection rates. J Knee Surg. 2023;36(4):354–61. https://doi.org/10.1055/s-0041-1733902.
3. Pannu TS, Villa JM, Corces A, Riesgo AM, Higuera CA. Synovial white blood cell count and differential to predict successful infection management in a two-stage revision. J Arthroplasty. 2022;37(6):1159–64. https://doi.org/10.1016/j.arth.2022.02.030.
4. Benda S, Mederake M, Schuster P, Fink B. Diagnostic value of C-reactive protein and serum white blood cell count during septic two-stage revision of total knee arthroplasties. Antibiotics (Basel). 2022;12(1):14. https://doi.org/10.3390/antibiotics12010014.
5. Logoluso N, Pellegrini A, Suardi V, Morelli I, Battaglia AG, D'Anchise R, et al. Can the leukocyte esterase strip test predict persistence of periprosthetic joint infection at second-stage reimplantation? J Arthroplasty. 2022;37(3):565–73. https://doi.org/10.1016/j.arth.2021.11.022.
6. Craig A, King SW, van Duren BH, Veysi VT, Jain S, Palan J. Articular spacers in two-stage revision arthroplasty for prosthetic joint infection of the hip and the knee. EFORT Open Rev. 2022;7(2):137–52. https://doi.org/10.1530/EOR-21-0037.
7. Fei Z, Zhang Z, Wang Y, Zhang H, Xiang S. Comparing the efficacy of articulating spacers in two-stage revision for periprosthetic joint infection following total knee arthroplasty: all-cement spacers vs sterilized replanted metal-polyethylene spacers. Int J Gen Med. 2022;15:3293–301. https://doi.org/10.2147/IJGM.S354808.
8. Russo A, Cavagnaro L, Chiarlone F, Alessio-Mazzola M, Felli L, Burastero G. Predictors of failure of two-stage revision in periprosthetic knee infection: a retrospective cohort study with a minimum two-year follow-up. Arch Orthop Trauma Surg. 2022;142(3):481–90. https://doi.org/10.1007/s00402-021-04265-5.
9. Hartman CW, Daubach EC, Richard BT, Lyden ER, Haider H, Kildow BJ, et al. Predictors of reinfection in prosthetic joint infections following two-stage reimplantation. J Arthroplasty. 2022;37(7S):S674–7. https://doi.org/10.1016/j.arth.2022.03.017.
10. Krizsan G, Sallai I, Veres DS, Prinz G, Szeker D, Skaliczki G. Rifampicin resistance and risk factors associated with significantly lower recovery rates after two-stage revision in patients with prosthetic joint infection. J Glob Antimicrob Resist. 2022;30:231–6. https://doi.org/10.1016/j.jgar.2022.06.020.
11. Kildow BJ, Springer BD, Brown TS, Lyden ER, Fehring TK, Garvin KL. Long term results of two-stage revision for chronic periprosthetic knee infection: a multicenter study. J Arthroplasty. 2022;37(6S):S327–32. https://doi.org/10.1016/j.arth.2022.01.029.
12. Kim DY, Seo YC, Kim CW, Lee CR, Jung SH. Factors affecting range of motion following two-stage revision arthroplasty for chronic periprosthetic knee infection. Knee Surg Relat Res. 2022;34(1):33. https://doi.org/10.1186/s43019-022-00162-2.
13. Lin YC, Lin YH, Chou JH, Lo YT, Chang CH, Lee SH, et al. Higher reinfection rate after two-stage revision arthroplasty in patients with refractory diabetes mellitus: a retrospective analysis with a minimum ten-year follow up. BMC Musculoskelet Disord. 2022;23(1):990. https://doi.org/10.1186/s12891-022-05964-9.

14. Qiao YJ, Li F, Zhang LD, Yu XY, Zhang HQ, Yang WB, et al. Analysis of the clinical efficacy of two-stage revision surgery in the treatment of periprosthetic joint infection in the knee: a retrospective study. World J Clin Cases. 2022;10(36):13239–49. https://doi.org/10.12998/wjcc.v10.i36.13239.
15. McPherson EJ, Tontz W Jr, Patzakis M, Woodsome C, Holton P, Norris L, et al. Outcome of infected total knee utilizing a staging system for prosthetic joint infection. Am J Orthop (Belle Mead NJ). 1999;28(3):161–5. PMID: 10195839.
16. Green CC, Valenzuela MM, Odum SM, Rowe TM, Springer BD, Fehring TK, et al. Hypoalbuminemia predicts failure of two-stage exchange for chronic periprosthetic joint infection of the hip and knee. J Arthroplasty. 2023;38(7):1363–8. https://doi.org/10.1016/j.arth.2023.01.012.
17. Theil C, Schneider KN, Gosheger G, Schmidt-Braekling T, Ackmann T, Dieckmann R, et al. Revision TKA with a distal femoral replacement is at high risk of reinfection after two-stage exchange for periprosthetic knee joint infection. Knee Surg Sports Traumatol Arthrosc. 2022;30(3):899–906. https://doi.org/10.1007/s00167-021-06474-2.
18. Charlson ME, Carrozzino D, Guidi J, Patierno C. Charlson comorbidity index: a critical review of clinimetric properties. Psychother Psychosom. 2022;91(1):8–35. https://doi.org/10.1159/000521288.
19. Chuang CA, Lee SH, Chang CH, Hu CC, Shih HN, Ueng SWN, et al. Application of structural allogenous bone graft in two-stage exchange arthroplasty for knee periprosthetic joint infection: a case control study. BMC Musculoskelet Disord. 2022;23(1):325. https://doi.org/10.1186/s12891-022-05228-6.
20. Christiner T, Yates P, Prosser G. Repeat two-stage revision for knee prosthetic joint infection results in very high failure rates. ANZ J Surg. 2022;92(3):487–92. https://doi.org/10.1111/ans.17446.
21. Steinicke AC, Schwarze J, Gosheger G, Moellenbeck B, Ackmann T, Theil C. Repeat two-stage exchange arthroplasty for recurrent periprosthetic hip or knee infection: what are the chances for success? Arch Orthop Trauma Surg. 2023;143(4):1731–40. https://doi.org/10.1007/s00402-021-04330-z.
22. Wignadasan W, Ibrahim M, Haddad FS. One- or two-stage reimplantation for infected total knee prosthesis? Orthop Traumatol Surg Res. 2023;109(1S):103453. https://doi.org/10.1016/j.otsr.2022.103453.
23. Lenguerrand E, Whitehouse MR, Kunutsor SK, Beswick AD, Baker RP, Rolfson O, et al.; National Joint Registry for England, Wales, Northern Ireland and the Isle of Man. Mortality and re-revision following single-stage and two-stage revision surgery for the management of infected primary knee arthroplasty in England and Wales: evidence from the National Joint Registry. Bone Joint Res. 2022;11(10):690–699. https://doi.org/10.1302/2046-3758.1110.BJR-2021-0555.R1.
24. Okafor CE, Nghiem S, Byrnes J. Is 2-stage septic revision worth the money? A cost-utility analysis of a 1-stage versus 2-stage septic revision of total knee arthroplasty. J Arthroplasty. 2023;38(2):347–54. https://doi.org/10.1016/j.arth.2022.09.003.

Revision Total Knee Arthroplasty for Arthrofibrosis

10

E. Carlos Rodríguez-Merchán

10.1 Introduction

Total knee arthroplasty (TKA) endures the gold standard for end-stage knee osteoarthritis. The frequency of stiffness after this procedure reported in literature varies from 1.3 to 5.3%. The causes of arthrofibrosis after TKA are multifactorial. Revision TKA (rTKA) is a successful technique when carried out for loosening, instability, mechanical implant failure, or infection. However, the outcomes of rTKA for idiopathic arthrofibrosis and stiffening are less favorable [1].

In 2021, Debbi et al. affirmed that stiffness after TKA is a challenging adverse event for both the patient and orthopedic surgeon, with a prevalence that ranges from 1 to 13%. There are several correctable mechanical causes for stiffness (Fig. 10.1). Idiopathic stiffness is frequently termed arthrofibrosis and is more difficult to manage. Once individuals have exhausted nonoperative options, including physical medicine and rehabilitation and manipulation under anesthesia (MUA), revision surgery might be considered [2].

The purpose of this chapter is to analyze recent literature on rTKA for arthrofibrosis.

E. C. Rodríguez-Merchán (✉)
Department of Orthopedic Surgery, La Paz University Hospital, Madrid, Spain

© The Author(s), under exclusive license to Springer Nature Switzerland AG 2024
E. C. Rodríguez-Merchán (ed.), *Advances in Revision Total Knee Arthroplasty*,
https://doi.org/10.1007/978-3-031-60445-4_10

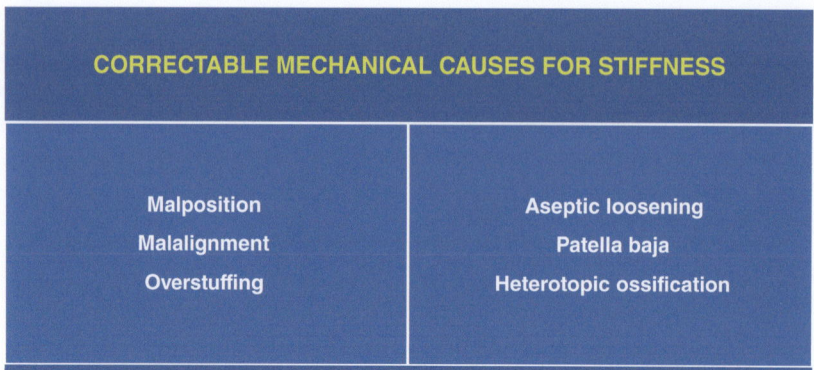

Fig. 10.1 Correctable mechanical causes for stiffness

10.2 Rotating-Hinge rTKA for Treatment of Serious Arthrofibrosis

In a study with level 3 of evidence published in 2019 by Bingham et al., they reported implant survivorship in individuals with arthrofibrosis revised with a rotating-hinge (RH) [3]. Thirty-four individuals revised with an RH for arthrofibrosis were matched to 68 individuals revised without an RH. The mean age was 63 years, 62% were female, mean body mass index (BMI) was 31 kg/m^2, and mean follow-up was 6 years. The mean range of motion (ROM) increased 20° (74°–94°) in the RH cohort versus 12° (87°–99°) in the non-RH cohort. Two MUAs were carried out in the RH cohort compared to nine in the non-RH cohort. Knee Society scores increased substantially in both cohorts. Survivorship free of revision for aseptic loosening at 10 years was 83% in the RH cohort versus 96% in the non-RH cohort. Survivorship free of any revision at 10 years was 54% in the RH cohort and 90% in the non-RH cohort. Forty percent of the revisions in the RH cohort were related to insert and bushing exchanges. Individuals with arthrofibrosis revised to an RH TKA had a 20° improvement in ROM, and MUA were half as common. However, there was a higher risk of re-revision in the RH cohort [3].

According to Debbie et al., RH rTKA has been demonstrated to be an efficacious surgical treatment for serious arthrofibrosis. They gave the following recommendations: accomplish appropriate exposure with a quadriceps snip; carry out a thorough synovectomy and debridement; make a balanced extension gap with a relatively loose flexion gap; distalize the joint line by resecting the additional proximal tibia in cases of patella baja; beware of refractory stiffness due to a scarred extensor mechanism; contemplate revising the patellar component; and consider carrying out a partial condylectomy at the medial and lateral distal aspects of the femur [2].

10.3 Hinged Versus CCK Revision Arthroplasty for the Stiff Total Knee

In 2019, Hermans et al. stated that it had been their perception that the poor outcomes in arthrofibrosis could be in part related to the employment of traditional posterior-stabilized (PS) or constrained condylar knee (CCK)-type revision implants [1]. They hypothesized that better outcomes could be accomplished in case a RH design is employed. The motive could be that RH designs permit for much more aggressive capsuloligament debridement and thereby more appropriate fibrosis removal, as long as assuring optimal implant stability, tibiofemoral rotational freedom, and flexion-extension space stability. They analyzed 40 individuals. Twenty-two received a hinged-type prosthetic device (18 Zimmer RH, four Stryker RH), and 18 received a less constrained condylar type prosthetic device (17 Legion CCK, one Vanguard CCK). Preoperative data were similar for RH as CCK-type implants except for knee pain score, which was substantially worse for the RH group (36 versus 44). At 2 years of follow-up, compared to CCK, the RH cohort exhibited substantially better postoperative outcomes for knee function scores (68.9 versus 54.2), knee function improvement (22.8 versus 4.8), knee pain improvement (26.4 versus 9.4), greater maximal flexion (99.9° versus 81.4°), better maximal extension (−1.9° versus −6.2°), greater flexion gain (35.8° versus 14.2°), and greater extension gain (8.6° vs 2°). This study showed that rTKA of the stiff knee employing a RH device can yield excellent outcomes in selected cases [1].

10.4 Arthrofibrosis After Primary TKA in Individuals with History of Hypertrophic Scar and Keloid Disorders

In a study with level 3 of evidence published in 2021 by Flick et al., they stated that arthrofibrosis endured one of the main causes for revision in primary TKA (pTKA). Similar in nature to arthrofibrosis, hypertrophic scars and keloid formation are a consequence of excessive collagen formation. They recognized and compared the percentages of postoperative adverse events related to arthrofibrosis after pTKA in individuals with history of hypertrophic scar and keloid disorders versus those without. Of 545,875 pTKAs, 11,461 (2.1%) had a keloid diagnosis at any time point in their record, while 534,414 (97.9%) had not. Individuals in the keloid group had a substantially higher association with ankylosis within 30 days, 90 days, 6 months, and 1 year after primary TKA. The keloid group also had a substantially greater risk of MUA. Individuals with keloids have increased odds risk of arthrofibrosis after pTKA. These individuals are subsequently at a higher odds risk of experiencing the procedures needed to manage arthrofibrosis, such as MUA and lysis of adhesions (LOA) [4].

10.5 Lysis of Adhesions for Arthrofibrosis After TKA Is Associated with Increased Risk of Subsequent rTKA

In a study with level 3 of evidence published in 2021 by Cregar et al., they analyzed the prevalence of LOA for postoperative arthrofibrosis after pTKA, and patient factors associated with LOA, and influence of LOA on rTKA. Individuals who experienced pTKA were identified in the Humana and Medicare databases. Individuals who experienced LOA within 1 year after TKA were defined as the "LOA" group. In total, 58,538 and 48,336 individuals experienced pTKA in the Medicare and Humana databases, respectively. Prevalence of LOA within 1 year after TKA was 0.56% in both databases. Age <75 years was a substantial predictor of LOA in both databases. Prevalence of rTKA was substantially higher for the "LOA" group when compared to the "TKA-only" group in both databases. LOA was the main predictor of rTKA within 2 years after index TKA in both databases. Besides, other factors were independently associated with increased odds of rTKA within 2 years after index TKA (Fig. 10.2). Prevalence of LOA after pTKA was low, with younger age being the main predictor for needing LOA. Individuals who experience LOA for arthrofibrosis within 1 year after pTKA have a significantly high risk for subsequent early rTKA [5].

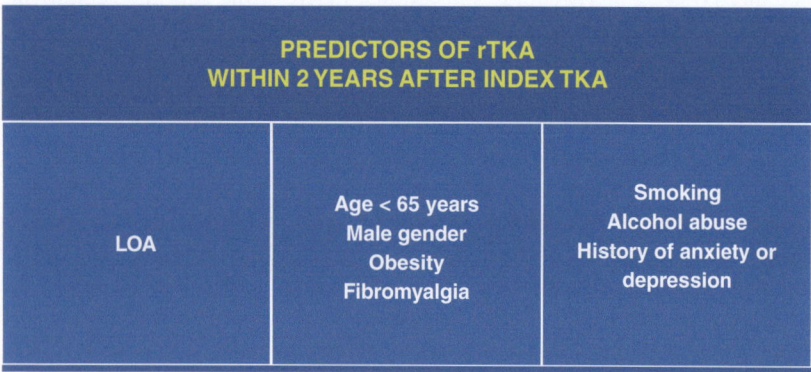

Fig. 10.2 Predictors of revision total knee arthroplasty (rTKA) within 2 years after index total knee arthroplasty (TKA). *LOA* lysis of adhesions (arthroscopy)

10.6 Individuals with Dupuytren's Contracture, Ledderhose Disease, and Peyronie's Disease Are at Higher Risk of Arthrofibrosis Following TKA

In 2021, Wang et al. tried to identify whether an association existed between Dupuytren's contracture, Ledderhose disease, and Peyronie's disease and arthrofibrosis after TKA. They compared the percentages of arthrofibrosis, MUA, LOA, and rTKA in individuals with independent chart diagnoses of Dupuytren's contracture, Ledderhose, or Peyronie's diseases versus those without. They found an increased odds risk of arthrofibrosis and MUA in individuals who have experienced TKA and had a diagnosis of Dupuytren's contracture, Ledderhose, or Peyronie's diseases [6].

10.7 MUA, Arthroscopic Lysis of Adhesions, or rTKA for Arthrofibrosis and Stiffness Following TKA

In 2022, Haffar et al. affirmed that there was no consensus regarding the optimal management for stiffness after TKA. A systematic review was carried out to compare the results of MUA, arthroscopic lysis of adhesions (aLOA), and rTKA for arthrofibrosis and stiffness following TKA. A total of 40 studies were included: 21 on rTKA, seven on aLOA, and 14 on MUA. The mean or median postoperative ROM was >90° in 6/20 (30%) rTKA, 5/7 (71%) aLOA, and 7/10 (70%) MUA studies. Postoperative Knee Society clinical and functional scores were the greatest in individuals who experienced MUA and aLOA. As many as 43% of rTKA individuals needed further care compared to 25% of aLOA and 17% of MUA individuals. Stiffness after TKA endures a challenging condition to treat. Nevertheless, current evidence suggests that individuals who experience rTKA have poorer clinical results and a greater need for further treatment compared to individuals who experience MUA or aLOA [7].

10.8 Results

In 2018, Ruhterford et al. assessed results following rTKA for arthrofibrosis. They analyzed 46 consecutive rTKAs for arthrofibrosis between 2007 and 2015 with minimum 2-year follow-up. Individuals were followed for a mean of 59 months. ROM and Knee Society scores significantly improved: with flexion improving from 88° to 103° and extension improving from 11° to 3°. There was not a relationship between patient or surgical factors and results. The rate of adverse events was 28.2% with a 17.4% reoperation rate. While revision for arthrofibrosis after TKA can be associated with substantial improvements in ROM and Knee Society scores, caution is advised given high percentages of revisions, reoperations, and adverse events. Thirty percent of individuals in this study had a reduction in one or more component of the Knee Society score or a net decrease in ROM after revision surgery [8].

In a study with level 4 of evidence published in 2023 by Rockov et al., they assessed ROM when rTKA was carried out for arthrofibrosis. They analyzed 42 TKAs diagnosed with arthrofibrosis with a minimum 2-year follow-up was performed. The primary outcome was ROM (flexion, extension, and total arc of motion) before and after rTKA, and secondary outcomes included patient-reported outcomes measurement information system (PROMIS) scores. The patient's pre-revision mean flexion was 85.6°, and mean extension was 10.1°. At the time of the revision, the mean age of the group was 64.7 years, the average BMI was 29.8, and 62% were female. At a mean follow-up of 4.5 years, rTKA substantially improved terminal flexion by 18.4°, terminal extension by 6.8°, and total arc of motion by 25.2°. The final ROM following rTKA was not substantially different from the patient's pre-primary TKA ROM. PROMIS physical function, depression, and pain interference scores were 39, 49, and 62, respectively. rTKA for arthrofibrosis substantially improved ROM at a mean follow-up of 4.5 years with over 25° of improvement in the total arc of motion, resulting in final ROM similar to pre-primary TKA ROM. Rockov et al. concluded that while physical medicine and rehabilitation and MUA endure the gold standard for the early management of stiffness following TKA, rTKA can improve ROM [9].

10.9 Conclusions

The prevalence of stiffness after TKA ranges from 1 to 13%. Once individuals have exhausted nonoperative options, including physical medicine and rehabilitation and MUA, revision surgery might be considered. The rate of adverse events after rTKA for arthrofibrosis is about 28%, while the reoperation rate is around 17%. When comparing the results of MUA, aLOA, and rTKA for arthrofibrosis and stiffness following TKA, as many as 43% of rTKA individuals need further care compared to 25% of aLOA and 17% of MUA individuals. Stiffness after TKA endures a challenging condition to treat. Nevertheless, current evidence suggests that individuals who experience rTKA have poorer clinical results and a greater need for further treatment compared to individuals who experience MUA or aLOA.

References

1. Hermans K, Vandenneucker H, Truijen J, Oosterbosch J, Bellemans J. Hinged versus CCK revision arthroplasty for the stiff total knee. Knee. 2019;26(1):222–7. https://doi.org/10.1016/j.knee.2018.10.012.
2. Debbi EM, Alpaugh K, Driscoll DA, Tarity TD, Gkiatas I, Sculco PK. Rotating hinge revision total knee arthroplasty for severe arthrofibrosis. JBJS Essent Surg Tech. 2021;11(4):e21.00009. https://doi.org/10.2106/JBJS.ST.21.00009.
3. Bingham JS, Bukowski BR, Wyles CC, Pareek A, Berry DJ, Abdel MP. Rotating-hinge revision total knee arthroplasty for treatment of severe arthrofibrosis. J Arthroplasty. 2019;34(7S):S271–6. https://doi.org/10.1016/j.arth.2019.01.072.

4. Flick TR, Wang CX, Patel AH, Hodo TW, Sherman WF, Sanchez FL. Arthrofibrosis after total knee arthroplasty: patients with keloids at risk. J Orthop Traumatol. 2021;22(1):1. https://doi.org/10.1186/s10195-020-00563-7.
5. Cregar WM, Khazi ZM, Lu Y, Forsythe B, Gerlinger TL. Lysis of adhesion for arthrofibrosis after total knee arthroplasty is associated with increased risk of subsequent revision total knee arthroplasty. J Arthroplasty. 2021;36(1):339–344.e1. https://doi.org/10.1016/j.arth.2020.07.018.
6. Wang CX, Flick TR, Patel AH, Sanchez F, Sherman WF. Patients with Dupuytren's contracture, Ledderhose disease, and Peyronie's disease are at higher risk of arthrofibrosis following total knee arthroplasty. Knee. 2021;29:190–200. https://doi.org/10.1016/j.knee.2021.02.009.
7. Haffar A, Goh GS, Fillingham YA, Torchia MT, Lonner JH. Treatment of arthrofibrosis and stiffness after total knee arthroplasty: an updated review of the literature. Int Orthop. 2022;46(6):1253–79. https://doi.org/10.1007/s00264-022-05344-x.
8. Rutherford RW, Jennings JM, Levy DL, Parisi TJ, Martin JR, Dennis DA. Revision total knee arthroplasty for arthrofibrosis. J Arthroplasty. 2018;33(7S):S177–81. https://doi.org/10.1016/j.arth.2018.03.037.
9. Rockov ZA, Byrne CT, Rezzadeh KT, Durst CR, Spitzer AI, Paiement GD, et al. Revision total knee arthroplasty for arthrofibrosis improves range of motion. Knee Surg Sports Traumatol Arthrosc. 2023;31(5):1859–64. https://doi.org/10.1007/s00167-023-07353-8.

Revision Total Knee Arthroplasty for Implant-Related Metal Allergy

E. Carlos Rodríguez-Merchán

11.1 Introduction

Hypersensitivity to implants is an uncommon adverse event of total knee arthroplasty (TKA). Metal can cause allergic symptomatology that if unresponsive to conservative management could lead to revision [1]. Conventional total knee arthroplasty (TKA), made of cobalt-based alloys, contains some metals that are skin sensitizers, such as nickel, chromium, cobalt, and molybdenum, so there is the possibility of a hypersensitivity reaction (metal allergy). In fact, 20–25% of individuals undergoing TKA acquire hypersensitivity to metals, but only less than 1% display symptoms (dermatitis, persistent painful synovitis of the knee, or aseptic loosening of the implant) [2]. The purpose of this chapter is to review recent knowledge on revision total knee arthroplasty (rTKA) for implant-related metal allergy.

11.2 Tests Utilized to Evaluate Metal Hypersensitivity

Skin patch testing (SPT) and lymphocyte transformation tests (LTT) are being habitually used to assess metal hypersensitivity. However, these tests are not completely reliable, and the majority of individuals are diagnosed on the basis of self-reported reactions [2].

E. C. Rodríguez-Merchán (✉)
Department of Orthopedic Surgery, La Paz University Hospital, Madrid, Spain

© The Author(s), under exclusive license to Springer Nature Switzerland AG 2024
E. C. Rodríguez-Merchán (ed.), *Advances in Revision Total Knee Arthroplasty*,
https://doi.org/10.1007/978-3-031-60445-4_11

11.2.1 Skin Patch Test (SPT)

In 2016, Bravo et al. stated that it was unclear whether a positive SPT for metal allergy in individuals with skin hypersensitivity to metals was associated with an increased risk of TKA failure. They aimed to determine whether individuals with a history of metal allergy who had a positive skin patch test (SPT+) had worse results following primary TKA compared with those with a negative skin patch test and compared with controls. Over 12 years, 127 individuals experienced 161 TKA after SPT (SPT; 56 were positive). Cases were matched by age, gender, body mass index (BMI), American Society of Anesthesiologists (ASA) score, implant type, and implant manufacturer to 161 control TKAs without any previous history of metal allergy and no SPT. Median follow-up was 5.3 years. Differences in outcome measures were evaluated between cohorts. Individuals with a SPT+ to metal did not have a higher adverse event, reoperation, or revision percentages compared with individuals with a SPT− and matched controls. Survivorship free of revision at 5 years was 98.1% for SPT+; 100% for SPT−; 97.6% for SPT+ controls, and 99% for SPT− controls. There was no statistically significant difference in postoperative pain between SPT+ and SPT− individuals and matched controls. In this study, a SPT+ for metals was of little practical value in forecasting the mid-run result following TKA [3].

11.2.2 Lymphocyte Transformation Test (LTT)

In a study with level 4 of evidence published in 2019 by Yang et al., they affirmed that the use of LTT had increased for diagnosing metal sensitivity associated with TKA, but its validity for the diagnosis of TKA failure due to an immune reaction had not been proven [4]. In the study, Yang et al. sought to characterize the relationship of a positive LTT result to histopathologic findings and clinical and functional results. They analyzed 27 well-fixed, aseptic, primary TKAs (pTKAs) in which the individual had continuous pain and/or stiffness and experienced revision TKA (rTKA) due to a suspected metal allergy to nickel, as determined on the basis of positive LTT. Periprosthetic tissue samples attained at the time of revision surgery were scored utilizing the aseptic lymphocyte-dominated vasculitis-associated lesion (ALVAL) scoring system [5]. Eight individuals were categorized as mildly reactive; eight individuals, moderately reactive; and 11 individuals, highly reactive to nickel by LTT. The prevailing findings on routine histopathologic analysis were fibrosis and varying grades of lymphocytic infiltration in 17 (63%) of the 27 cases. The average ALVAL score of the group was 3.1 of a maximum score of 10. Average Knee Society Score (KSS) values improved post-revision, as did range of motion (ROM). On the basis of this analysis, including histopathologic evaluation, LTT results alone were insufficient for the diagnosis of TKA failure due to an immune reaction. A positive LTT might not indicate that an immune reaction is the source of pain and stiffness post-TKA [4].

According to Malahias et al. (2023), LTT is frequently utilized in the workup for potential metal allergy after TKA, but the correlation of this test with other diagnostic metal allergy findings in individuals experiencing rTKA for suspected metal allergy has not been determined [6]. Nineteen TKAs in which both components were revised for presumed implant-related metal allergy based on history, physical, and LTT testing, to nonnickel-containing implants, were analyzed. Histopathologic samples obtained intraoperatively were semiquantitatively analyzed utilizing both the Hospital for Special Surgery (HSS) synovial pathology score and the ALVAL score [5]. As histopathology control cohort, Malahias et al. included in the study an additional group of 17 individuals who underwent rTKA and had no history of reported or tested metal sensitivity. All preoperative LTT results were highly reactive to nickel. However, this did not correlate with local periarticular tissue response in 18 of 19 cases which exhibited a low HSS synovial score (mean, 3.8; of a maximum score of 28) and the low ALVAL scores (mean, 2.5/10; of a maximum score of 10). There were no any substantial differences between the study cohort (suspected implant-related metal allergy) and the control cohort (nonsuspected implant-related metal allergy) in regard to (1) the ALVAL score and (2) the HSS synovial inflammatory score. Knee Society Clinical Rating System (KSCRS) function score improved substantially after rTKA (mean postoperative increase, 34), as well as mean visual analog scale (VAS) pain (mean postoperative decrease, 33.3) score. The short-run survival percentage (at mean follow-up of 26.1 months) of this patient group was 100%. In this group of revised TKA individuals with suspected nickel allergy based on clinical presentation and LTT positive results, intraoperative histopathology was basically normal. However, all individuals with suspected nickel allergy exhibited a substantial clinical and functional improvement with excellent short-run survival percentages [6].

11.3 Clinical Results of rTKA in Individuals with Presumed Metal Allergy

In 2017, Stathopoulos et al. reported the case of an individual with generalized pruritus and metal taste beginning during the first postoperative month following TKA. Dermal allergy exams demonstrated that the individual had hypersensitivity to nickel sulfate and cobalt chloride and bone cement. Conservative management with antihistamine medication and corticosteroids failed to control the symptoms. The individual experienced rTKA with a hypoallergic prosthesis 8 months after the primary procedure. Complete disappearance of the symptoms happened 3 months after revision. The latest follow-up assessment (3 years post-revision) was unremarkable. Stathopoulos et al. stated that an exhaustive medical history should be attained from every candidate for TKA, and in cases of previous serious allergic reactions to metals, plastics, or glues, SPT of the components of the future prosthesis should be performed. When an already implanted prosthesis causes symptoms like pain, edema, pruritus, erythema, limited ROM, and increase in joint's temperature, the likelihood of allergy to metals and/or bone cement (in case of cemented prosthesis) should be checked after the exclusion of other causes like infection. If symptoms cannot be controlled by conservative treatment, rTKA should be decided and performed with hypoallergic prosthesis [1].

According to Whiteside (2022), metal and cement allergy affects a small subset of individuals, causing intense pain and often systemic reaction after TKA. Revision with ceramic-surfaced femoral components has been described to solve these symptoms of metal allergy, but no solution was available for individuals with allergies to metal and bone cement. Five individuals (five knees) with proven metal allergy were revised with custom porous-coated ceramic femoral components (magnesia-stabilized zirconia). Inclusion criteria included the history of clinically established serious metal allergy, intense pain, swelling, and effusion >1 year following TKA, negative workup for infection, loosening, and ligament imbalance. Mean KSS for all five individuals revised with custom cementless ceramic femoral components improved substantially for objective score (preoperative, 39; most recent visit, 90) and function score (preoperative, 33; most recent visit 93). The conclusion was that individuals who are allergic both to metals and bone cement would be candidates solely for porous-coated ceramic implants fixed without bone cement [7].

In a study with level 4 of evidence published in 2022 by Bulaïd et al., they stated that rTKA for suspicion of metal hypersensitivity might need hypoallergenic implants [8]. They evaluated short-run outcomes and survival of rTKA for metal hypersensitivity utilizing a multilayer implant coating. Their hypothesis was that multilayer implant coating improves functional outcomes in rTKA, with survival comparable to primary coated implants. A single-center retrospective observational study included 28 patients (30 knees) experiencing rTKA for metal hypersensitivity utilizing a coated implant. Exclusion criteria included implant malpositioning and history of infection in the affected knee. Clinical and radiological outcomes were evaluated on the International Knee Society (IKS) [9] and SF-36 functional scores [10] and Ewald radiological score [11]. Survival was calculated on Kaplan-Meier estimation [12]. Mean follow-up was 3.8 years. Mean IKS score increased by 40.2 points (40%). Mean ROM increased by 17°. Mean physical and mental SF-36 components were, respectively, 44.7 and 46.1. Survivorship was 93%. There was substantial functional improvement after rTKA for metal hypersensitivity. There were no short-run adverse events related to the zirconium nitrate coating [8].

In 2022, Bracey et al. affirmed that metal allergy testing may impact clinical decision-making for individuals experiencing a TKA [13]. They compared different metal allergy test outcomes and clinical results following primary TKA (pTKA) and rTKA in individuals with and without metal hypersensitivity. pTKA ($N = 28$) and rTKA ($N = 20$) TKA individuals undergoing hypoallergenic implants for metal allergies diagnosed by SPT, lymphocyte proliferation testing (LPT), or LTT were retrospectively reviewed. Postoperative clinical results of these individuals were compared to those of individuals without metal hypersensitivity matched by age, BMI, gender, and follow-up duration. SPT and LPT exhibited weak agreement for nickel and minimal agreement for cobalt. SPT and LTT exhibited minimal agreement for nickel; weak agreement for titanium, bone cement, vanadium, and zirconium; but strong agreement for chromium and cobalt. LPT and LTT agreement was weak. Compared to matched controls, metal hypersensitivity individuals experiencing pTKAs with hypoallergenic implants showed less improvement in KSS, Veterans RAND 12 physical component scores [14], and ROM. Bracey et al. concluded that individuals experiencing rTKAs for multiple indications including metal hypersensitivity had worse clinical results with substantially worse improvements in Knee Society functional scores (KSFS) compared to matched controls. Metal allergy tests yield conflicting outcomes. Hypersensitivity individuals might experience inferior clinical results even with hypoallergenic implants [13].

11.4 Practical Approach to Metal Hypersensitivity in TKA Individuals

According to Rodríguez-Merchán and Liddle, most individuals with metal allergy tolerate the conventional implants without adverse events; and some authors suggest that there is no reason for using a "hypoallergenic" TKA in individuals with skin sensitivity to metals. However, considering the controversy over whether or not to utilize a conventional pTKA in individuals who report having a metal allergy, the logical decision is to utilize a "hypoallergenic" primary prosthesis (Figs. 11.1 and 11.2). There are two "hypoallergenic" alternatives: (1) equivalent design but with different materials (oxidized zirconium, ceramic, or titanium-based alloys); (2) equivalent designs but with coatings, normally titanium niobium or titanium nitride (Tables 11.1 and 11.2). In individuals in whom a conventional pTKA fails due to metal hypersensitivity, a "hypoallergenic" rTKA should be recommended. However, before performing it, it is advisable to carry out knee arthroscopy to get tissue for microbiological and histopathological studies to exclude infection [2].

In a scoping review published in 2021 by Matar et al., they stated that evidence indicated that metal hypersensitivity was an uncommon adverse event with some histopathological features leading to pain and dissatisfaction with no dependable screening tests preoperatively. According to Matar et al., hypoallergenic implants are viable alternatives for individuals with self-reported/confirmed metal hypersensitivity if declared preoperatively; however, concerns remain over their long-run results with ceramic implants outperforming titanium nitride-coated implants. For individuals presenting with painful TKA, metal hypersensitivity is a diagnosis of exclusion where SPT, LTT, and synovial biopsies are useful adjuncts prior to revision surgery is undertaken to hypoallergenic implants [15].

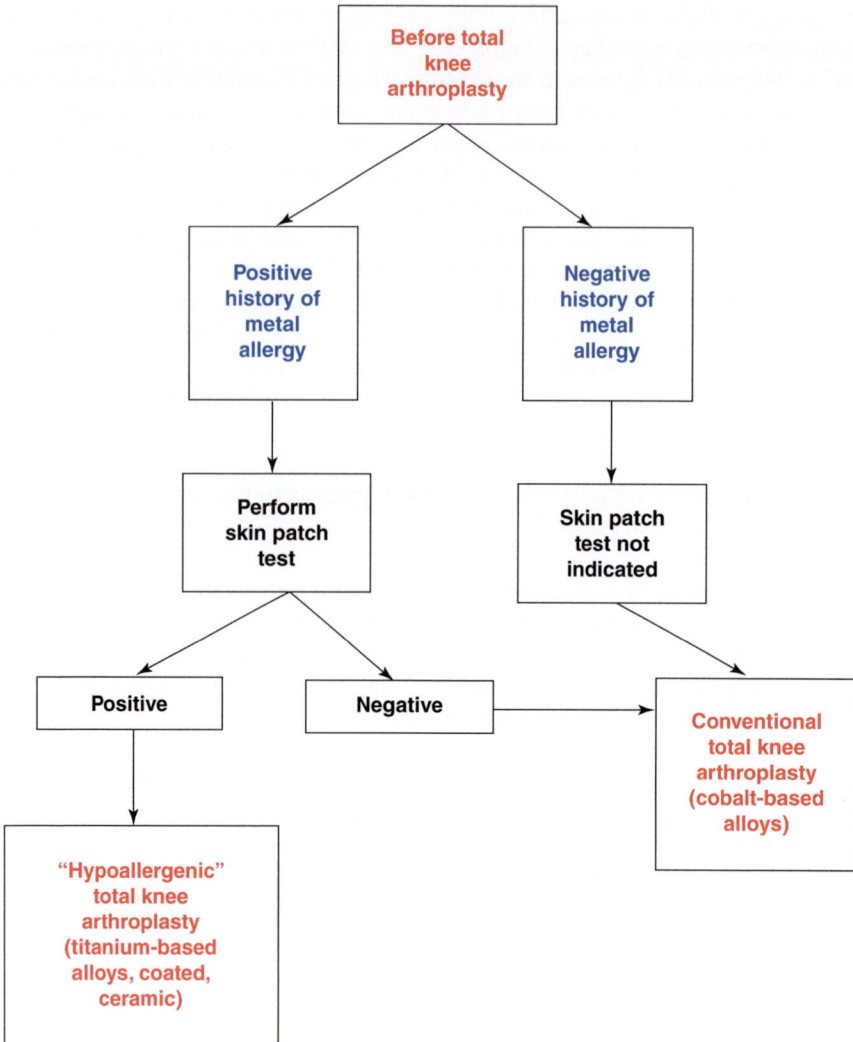

Fig. 11.1 Algorithm for the selection of individuals who will need a hypoallergenic primary total knee arthroplasty (pTKA)

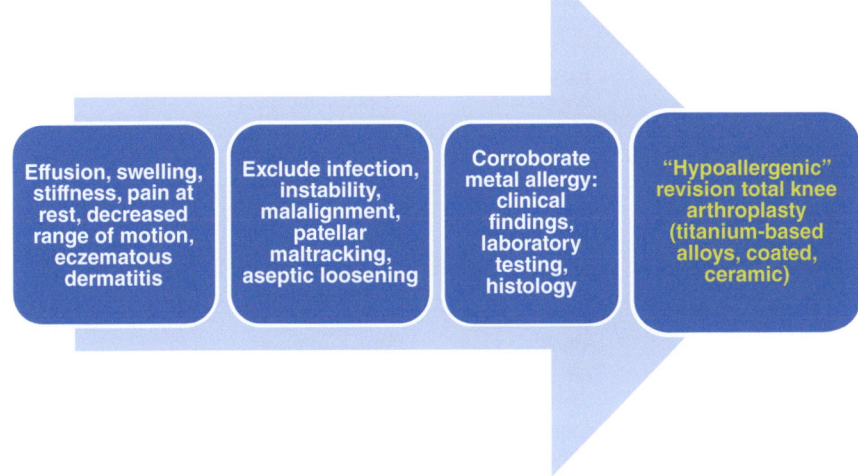

Fig. 11.2 Algorithm for the diagnosis and management of metal allergy-related adverse events following conventional primary total knee arthroplasty (pTKA)

Table 11.1 Noncoated metal "hypersensitivity-friendly" primary total knee arthroplasties (pTKAs)

Implant manufacturer	TKA system	Femoral component	Tibial component	Same design and instrumentation as the conventional system
Smith & Nephew	Genesis II	Oxinium oxidized zirconium (accessible off the shelf)	Titanium	Yes
Smith & Nephew	Genesis II	Oxinium oxidized zirconium (accessible off the shelf)	All-Poly® tibial (made entirely of polyethylene without metal back)	Yes
Smith & Nephew	Legion primary	Oxinium oxidized zirconium (accessible off the shelf)	Titanium	Yes
Zimmer	NexGen	Titanium (accessible off the shelf)	Titanium (accessible off the shelf)	Yes

pTKA primary total knee arthroplasty

Table 11.2 Coated metal "hypersensitivity-friendly" primary total knee arthroplasties (pTKAs)

Implant manufacturer	TKA system	Femoral component	Tibial component	Same design and instrumentation as the conventional system
B. Braun & Aesculap	Columbus AS implant system	Complete zirconia nitride coating of the standard implant (accessible off the shelf)	Complete zirconia nitride coating of the standard implant (accessible off the shelf)	Yes
Biomet	Vanguard	Complete titanium niobium nitride coating of Vanguard knee (accessible off the shelf)	Complete titanium niobium nitride coating of Vanguard knee (accessible off the shelf)	Yes
Depuy	PFC Sigma	Complete titanium nitride coated (custom-made)	Complete titanium nitride coated (custom-made)	Yes
Stryker	Triathlon	Complete titanium nitride coated (accessible off the shelf)	Complete titanium nitride coated (accessible off the shelf)	Yes

pTKA primary total knee arthroplasty

11.5 Conclusions

Between 20 and 25% of individuals undergoing TKA acquire hypersensitivity to metals, but only less than 1% display symptoms (dermatitis, persistent painful synovitis of the knee, or aseptic loosening of the implant). For individuals presenting with painful TKA, metal hypersensitivity is a diagnosis of exclusion where SPT, LTT, and synovial biopsies are useful adjuncts prior to revision surgery is undertaken to hypoallergenic implants. In individuals in whom a conventional pTKA fails due to metal hypersensitivity, a "hypoallergenic" rTKA should be recommended. However, before performing it, it is advisable to carry out knee arthroscopy to get tissue for microbiological and histopathological studies to exclude infection.

References

1. Stathopoulos IP, Andrianopoulos N, Paschaloglou D, Tsarouchas I. Revision total knee arthroplasty due to bone cement and metal hypersensitivity. Arch Orthop Trauma Surg. 2017;137(2):267–71. https://doi.org/10.1007/s00402-016-2614-6.
2. Rodríguez-Merchán EC, Liddle AD. Total knee arthroplasty in patients with a history of metal allergy: conventional implant or hypoallergenic implant? In: Rodríguez-Merchán EC, Liddle AD, editors. Controversies in orthopedic surgery of the lower limbs. Cham: Springer Nature Switzerland AG; 2021. p. 151–60.

3. Bravo D, Wagner ER, Larson DR, Davis MP, Pagnano MW, Sierra RJ. No increased risk of knee arthroplasty failure in patients with positive skin patch testing for metal hypersensitivity: a matched cohort study. J Arthroplasty. 2016;31(8):1717–21. https://doi.org/10.1016/j.arth.2016.01.024.
4. Yang S, Dipane M, Lu CH, Schmalzried TP, McPherson EJ. Lymphocyte transformation testing (LTT) in cases of pain following total knee arthroplasty: little relationship to histopathologic findings and revision outcomes. J Bone Joint Surg Am. 2019;101(3):257–64. https://doi.org/10.2106/JBJS.18.00134.
5. Campbell P, Shimmin A, Walter L, Solomon M. Metal sensitivity as a cause of groin pain in metal-on-metal hip resurfacing. J Arthroplasty. 2008;23(7):1080–5. https://doi.org/10.1016/j.arth.2007.09.024.
6. Malahias MA, Bauer TW, Manolopoulos PP, Sculco PK, Westrich GH. Allergy testing has no correlation with intraoperative histopathology from revision total knee arthroplasty for implant-related metal allergy. J Knee Surg. 2023;36(1):6–17. https://doi.org/10.1055/s-0041-1729618.
7. Whiteside LA. Clinical results of revision TKA in patients with presumed metal and cement allergy. J Arthroplasty. 2022;37(6S):S250–7. https://doi.org/10.1016/j.arth.2022.02.052.
8. Bulaïd Y, Djebara AE, Belhaouane R, Havet E, Dehl M, Mertl P. Beneficial effect of a zirconium-nitride-coated implant in total knee arthroplasty revision for suspected metal hypersensitivity. Orthop Traumatol Surg Res. 2022;108(5):103320. https://doi.org/10.1016/j.otsr.2022.103320.
9. Insall JN, Dorr LD, Scorr RD, Scott WN. Rationale of the knee society clinical rating system. Clin Orthop Relat Res. 1989;248:13–4. PMID: 2805470.
10. Saris-Baglama RN, Dewey CJ, Chisholm GB, et al. QualityMetric health outcomes™ scoring software 4.0. Lincoln: QualityMetric Incorporated; 2010. p. 138.
11. Ewald FC. The knee society total knee arthroplasty roentgenographic evaluation and scoring system. Clin Orthop Relat Res. 1989;248:9–12. PMID: 2805502.
12. Kaplan EL, Meier P. Nonparametric estimation from incomplete observations. J Am Stat Assoc. 1958;53(282):457–81.
13. Bracey DN, Hegde V, Johnson R, Kleeman-Forsthuber L, Jennings J, Dennis D. Poor correlation among metal hypersensitivity testing modalities and inferior patient-reported outcomes after primary and revision total knee arthroplasties. Arthroplast Today. 2022;18:138–42. https://doi.org/10.1016/j.artd.2022.09.016.
14. Iqbal SU, Rogers W, Selim A, Qian S, Lee A, Ren XS, et al. The Veterans Rand 12 item health survey (VR-12): what it is and how it is used. Boston University. pp 1–12. https://www.bu.edu/sph/files/2015/01/veterans_rand_12_item_health_survey_vr-12_2007.pdf. Accessed 22 June 2023.
15. Matar HE, Porter PJ, Porter ML. Metal allergy in primary and revision total knee arthroplasty: a scoping review and evidence-based practical approach. Bone Jt Open. 2021;2(10):785–95. https://doi.org/10.1302/2633-1462.210.BJO-2021-0098.R1.

Robotic-Assisted Revision Total Knee Arthroplasty

12

E. Carlos Rodríguez-Merchán, Carlos A. Encinas-Ullán, Juan S. Ruiz-Pérez, and Primitivo Gómez-Cardero

12.1 Introduction

During the past decades, robotic-assisted technology has underwent an extraordinary progress in the discipline of total knee arthroplasty (TKA) and has shown promise in improving the accuracy and precision of implantation and alignment in primary TKA (pTKA) [1]. Robotic-assisted pTKA (RA-pTKA) diminishes the surgical time, inpatient length of stay (LOS), as well as 90-day complication and readmission rates of complex pTKA to the level of noncomplex pTKA. Greater case complexity does not appear to have a negative influence on economic outcome parameters when surgery is carried out with robotic assistance [2].

The results of the study of Adamska et al. suggest satisfactory outcomes after both RA-pTKA methods and manual pTKA (M-pTKA). RA-pTKA and M-pTKA stand for a safe and dependable management method for osteoarthritis. Patients reported excellent relief in functional results, and the radiological outcomes showed that the better precision does not necessarily result in a better outcome. Therefore, RA-pTKA does not imply strong enough pros in comparison to the manual technique, especially in terms of cost-efficiency and surgical time [3].

Regarding revision TKA (rTKA), it endures a technically challenging technique with issues of large-scale osseous defects and damage to nearby anatomical structures. Therefore, orthopedic surgeons are trying to employ the capabilities of robotic-assisted technology for rTKA [1]. According to Paisner et al., Black individuals have lower percentages of RA-TKA compared to White, Asian, and Hispanic individuals [4]. The purpose of this chapter is to describe recent advances on RA-rTKA.

E. C. Rodríguez-Merchán (✉) · C. A. Encinas-Ullán · J. S. Ruiz-Pérez · P. Gómez-Cardero
Department of Orthopedic Surgery, La Paz University Hospital, Madrid, Spain

© The Author(s), under exclusive license to Springer Nature Switzerland AG 2024
E. C. Rodríguez-Merchán (ed.), *Advances in Revision Total Knee Arthroplasty*, https://doi.org/10.1007/978-3-031-60445-4_12

12.2 Recent Advances on Robotic-Assisted rTKA (RA-rTKA)

Steelman et al. reported a case in which robotic-assisted method was utilized to revise a failed pTKA. In this case, a revision implant system was used with both femoral and tibial cones and medial and lateral posterior femoral augments. They were able to carry out very small fresh cuts with robot arm assisted and adjust the posterior femoral cut to put augments both medially and laterally [5].

In 2021, MacAskill et al. related a case report in which they utilized robotic-assisted technology in rTKA. They affirmed that robotic assistance during rTKA might improve component alignment and increase prosthesis lifespan. They concluded that future studies were required to explore the impact on prosthesis longevity and expenditure [6].

In 2023, Ngim et al. stated that rTKA was a challenging technique and that the robotic-assisted system had demonstrated to increase the precision of preoperative planning and improve reproducibility in pTKA. In their report, they related the surgical procedure for RA-rTKA and the possible benefits of this procedure. They analyzed 19 individuals. Inclusion criteria were individuals who had Mako™ RA-rTKA performed within the study period with a more than 6 months of follow-up. All 19 individuals were followed up for 6–18 months. All individuals in this report had good recoveries without requiring any re-revision surgery. Ngim et al. concluded that with the development of dedicated revision total knee software, RA-rTKA can be a promising procedure that might improve surgical results by increasing the precision of implant placement and soft tissue protection and accomplishing a better well-balanced knee [7].

In a scoping review published in 2023 by Xu et al., they stated that current accessible information suggests that robotic-assisted technology might help orthopedic surgeons to reproducibly carry out preoperative plans and accurately accomplish operative targets during rTKA [1]. Figures 12.1 and 12.2 show two currently used RA-TKA techniques.

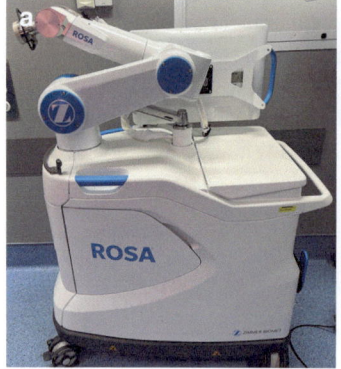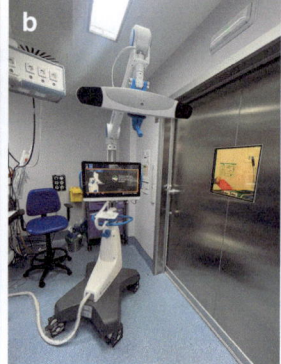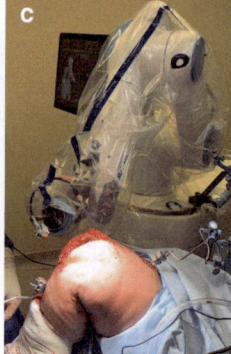

Fig. 12.1 (**a–c**) ROSA robotic-assisted total knee arthroplasty (RA-TKA) (Zimmer Biomet, Warsaw, IN, USA): (**a**) ROSA robot arm; (**b**) ROSA robot camera and monitor to be positioned in front of the surgeon; (**c**) ROSA robot arm positioning the cutting guide

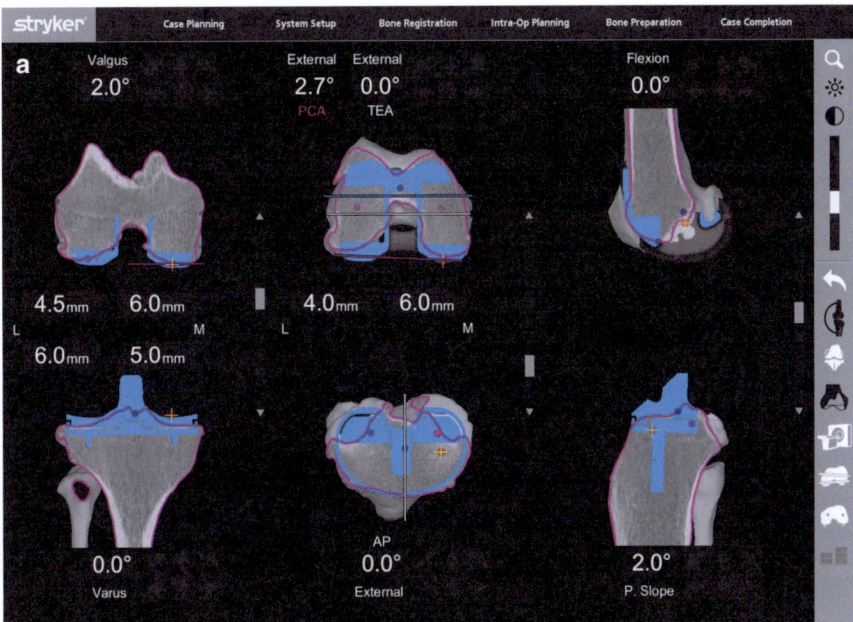

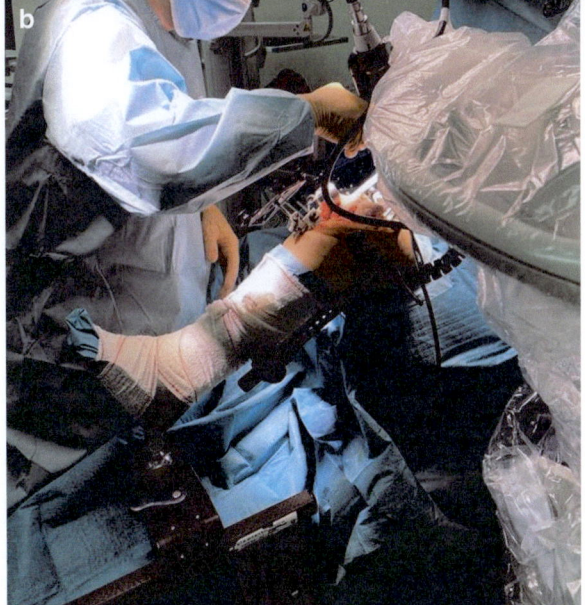

Fig. 12.2 (**a**, **b**) MAKO-assisted total knee arthroplasty (TKA) (MAKO Surgical Corporation [Stryker], Fort Lauderdale, FL, USA): (**a**) preoperative implant planning; (**b**) cutting with robot arm

12.3 Benefits and Risks of Robotic-Assisted rTKA (RA-rTKA)

For RA-rTKA, the benefits primarily include accurate bone cutting and the capability to locate the component alignment and mechanical alignment, which is frequently a challenge due to the loss of osseous reference points after implant removal. However, robotic-assisted technology needs preoperative computed tomography (CT) scan data, which have long been a concern raised as to the possible harm related to radiation exposure (e.g., 0.16 mSv for standard knee CT and 4.8 mSv for Makoplasty protocol) [6]. Figure 12.3 summarizes the main pros and cons of RA-rTKA.

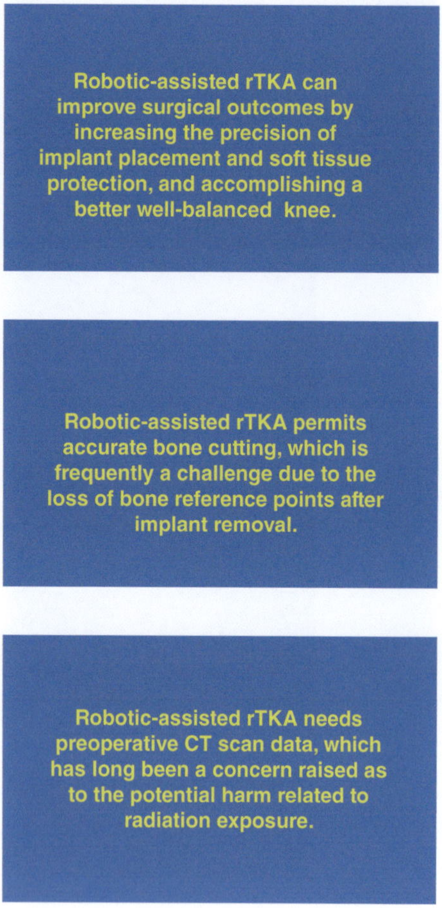

Fig. 12.3 Pros and cons of robotic-assisted revision total knee arthroplasty (RA-rTKA). *CT* computed tomography

- Robotic-assisted rTKA can improve surgical outcomes by increasing the precision of implant placement and soft tissue protection, and accomplishing a better well-balanced knee.
- Robotic-assisted rTKA permits accurate bone cutting, which is frequently a challenge due to the loss of bone reference points after implant removal.
- Robotic-assisted rTKA needs preoperative CT scan data, which has long been a concern raised as to the potential harm related to radiation exposure.

12.4 Conclusion

The current knowledge confirms the feasibility of robotic-assisted technology in rTKA, which may help orthopedic surgeons to carry out preoperative plans and accurately accomplish operative targets. However, concerns remain regarding further osseous loss after implant removal, and whether robotic-assisted surgery will improve implant placement and long-run survivorship, so further research is warranted.

References

1. Wu XD, Zhou Y, Shao H, Yang D, Guo SJ, Huang W. Robotic-assisted revision total joint arthroplasty: a state-of-the-art scoping review. EFORT Open Rev. 2023;8(1):18–25. https://doi.org/10.1530/EOR-22-0105.
2. Stauss R, Savov P, Tuecking LR, Windhagen H, Ettinger M. Robotic-assisted TKA reduces surgery duration, length of stay and 90-day complication rate of complex TKA to the level of noncomplex TKA. Arch Orthop Trauma Surg. 2023;143(6):3423–30. https://doi.org/10.1007/s00402-022-04618-8.
3. Adamska O, Modzelewski K, Szymczak J, Świderek J, Maciąg B, Czuchaj P, et al. Robotic-assisted total knee arthroplasty utilizing NAVIO, CORI imageless systems and manual TKA accurately restore femoral rotational alignment and yield satisfactory clinical outcomes: a randomized controlled trial. Medicina (Kaunas). 2023;59(2):236. https://doi.org/10.3390/medicina59020236.
4. Paisner ND, Upfill-Brown AM, Donnelly PC, De A, Sassoon AA. Racial disparities in rates of revision and use of modern features in total knee arthroplasty: a national registry study. J Arthroplasty. 2023;38(3):464–469.e3. https://doi.org/10.1016/j.arth.2022.09.023.
5. Steelman K, Carlson K, Ketner A. Utilization of robotic arm assistance for revision of primary total knee arthroplasty: a case report. J Orthop Case Rep. 2021;11(8):50–4. https://doi.org/10.13107/jocr.2021.v11.i08.2362.
6. MacAskill M, Blickenstaff B, Caughran A, Bullock M. Revision total knee arthroplasty using robotic arm technology. Arthroplast Today. 2021;13:35–42. https://doi.org/10.1016/j.artd.2021.11.003.
7. Ngim HJ, Van Bavel D, De Steiger R, Tang AWW. Robotic-assisted revision total knee arthroplasty: a novel surgical technique. Arthroplasty. 2023;5(1):5. https://doi.org/10.1186/s42836-022-00160-5.

Metal Augments, Polyethylene Thickness, and Stem Length Affect Tibial Baseplate Load Transfer in Revision Total Knee Arthroplasty

E. Carlos Rodríguez-Merchán

13.1 Introduction

According to Lamonica et al. (2023), it is not known how metal augments, polyethylene (PE) liner thickness, and length of cemented stem contribute to load transfer when reconstructing uncontained tibial metaphyseal bone loss of Anderson Orthopaedic Research Institute (AORI) type II defects during revision total knee arthroplasty (rTKA) (Fig. 13.1). They analyzed the influence of these three variables on load transfer through the tibial baseplate. For a fixed defect depth, they hypothesized that there is a combination of liner and augment thickness and stem length that reduces bone stress, diminishing the risk of aseptic loosening. They performed a finite element analysis (FEA) to model stresses at the bone-cement interface with different iterations of metal augments, PE liner thicknesses, and fully cemented stems lengths. For a 20-mm tibial defect, constructs with thicker metal augments and thinner PE liners were better. Constructs with a fully cemented stem further diminished bone stress on the tibial plateau. Bone stress was lowest when a 100-mm fully cemented stem was utilized, while stems between 30 and 80 mm gave similar outcomes. The conclusion was that when addressing a tibial bone defect of AORI type II in rTKA, this FEA model showed that surgeons should opt to utilize the thickest metal augments in combination with a fully cemented stem with an added length of at least 30 mm, which permits for surgical flexibility together with the most stable construct. This study was remarkably limited by lack of modeling of knee joint moments, which are important when deeming micromotion, bone-implant interface, and stem efficacy [1].

The purpose of this chapter is to revise recent developments on how metal augments, PE thickness, and stem length affect tibial baseplate load transfer in rTKA.

E. C. Rodríguez-Merchán (✉)
Department of Orthopedic Surgery, La Paz University Hospital, Madrid, Spain

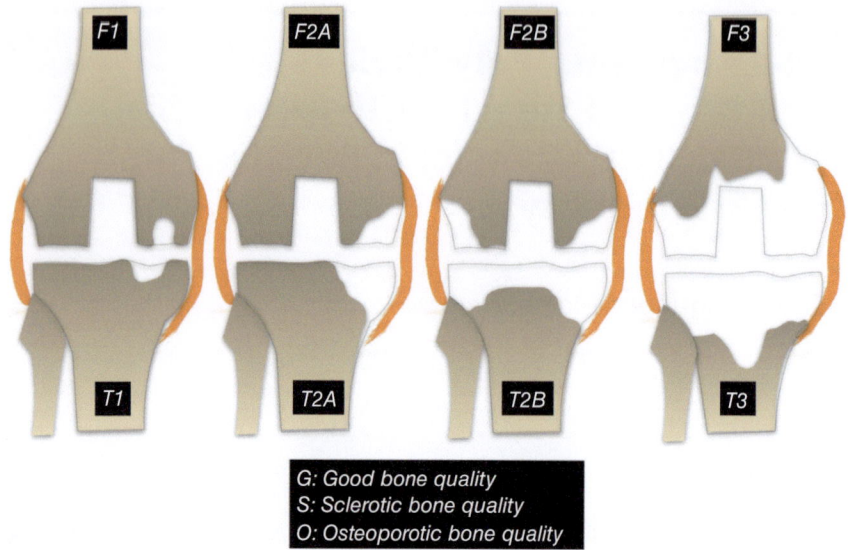

Fig. 13.1 Anderson Orthopaedic Research Institute (AORI) radiographic classification system for bone loss in patients undergoing revision total knee arthroplasty (rTKA)

13.2 Metal Augments

In 2016, Sculco et al. stated that the treatment of bone loss in rTKA had evolved over the past decade. While the management of small- to moderate-sized defects had shown good outcomes with a variety of traditional techniques (cement and screws, small metal augments, impaction bone grafting, or modular stems), the management of severe defects continued to be difficult. The utilization of a structural allograft had decreased in recent years because of an increased failure percentage with long-run follow-up and with the introduction of highly porous metal augments that emphasized biological metaphyseal fixation. Reported mid-run outcomes on the utilization of tantalum cones in individuals with severe bone loss had reaffirmed the success of this management approach [2].

In 2018, Innocenti et al. affirmed that augments were a common solution for managing bone loss in rTKA and the industry was rendering to orthopedic surgeons several alternatives, in terms of material, thickness, and shapes. In reality, while the election of the shape and the thickness was chiefly dictated by the osseous defect, no proper guidelines were available to select the optimal material for a specific clinical situation. Nonetheless, different materials could induce different osseous responses and, later, potentially compromise implant stability and performances. They performed a biomechanical analysis by means of finite element modeling about existing features for augment designs. The following augment features were analyzed: position (distal/proximal and posterior), thickness (5, 10, and 15 mm), and material (bone cement, porous metal, and solid metal). For all analyzed configurations, bone stresses were studied in different regions and compared among all configurations and the control model for which no augments were utilized. Outcomes demonstrated that the utilization of any kind of augment generally induces a change in bone stresses, especially in the region close to the bone cut. The porous metal was considered as a good alternative for defects of any size [3].

According to Rajgopal et al. (2021), managing severe periarticular bone loss poses a great defiance in complex primary total knee arthroplasty (pTKA) and rTKA. Impaction bone graft, structural allografts, metal augments, and megaprosthesis are some of the approaches utilized to address major bone loss. Tantalum metal cones (Zimmer, Warsaw, IN) were introduced as an alternative to manage this group of individuals. The pros of these cones include very good biocompatibility, high porosity with osteoconductive potential, and a modulus of elasticity between cortical and cancellous bone. Besides, it is bioactive and offers an intrinsically high friction fit. A group of 62 individuals with severe distal femoral and proximal tibial bone loss were operated for pTKA and rTKA between January 2007 and December 2014 and followed up for a mean period of 108.5 months. Preoperative and postoperative range of motion (ROM) and Knee Society score (KSS) were documented. Postoperatively, long leg X-rays were taken at each follow-up visit to determine osteointegration, evidence of loosening, and migration. The ROM and KSS improved considerably from preoperative a value of 63.9° and 52 to 102.1° and 76.1, respectively, at the final follow-up visit in the primary group and 52.14° and 38.1 to 92° and 68.5, respectively, in the revision group. Serial radiographs showed full osteointegration of the tantalum metal cones at the final follow-up. This study showed very good mid-run survivorship of tantalum metal cones with foreseeable osteointegration and good results (clinical and radiological) in management of severe femoral and tibial metaphyseal bone defects in complex pTKAs and rTKAs [4].

In 2021, Jacquet et al. compared the functional results and implant survivorship at a minimum of 5 years of follow-up of several reconstruction methods with or without metaphyseal cone and stems of variable length. A retrospective comparative matched analysis was carried out from two prospectively collected databases. Only individuals who experienced rTKA procedures for aseptic causes utilizing a single design of rotating hinge knee with a minimum of 5 years of follow-up were analyzed. Individuals were separated into three cohorts: trabecular metal (TM) cones + short cemented stems (TM + short stem [SS]), TM cones + long uncemented stems (TM + long stem [LS]), and no cone (NC) + long uncemented stems (NC + LS). A matching process based on age (±5 years) was realized. Ninety-nine individuals were included: 33 in the TM + SS group, 33 in the TM + LS group, and 33 in the NC + LS group. The mean time of follow-up was 9.3 years. A substantial difference of the improvement of subscale pain, symptom, activities of daily living, quality of life of the Knee Injury and Osteoarthritis Outcome Score, and knee function of the KSS was found in favor of TM + SS cohort compared with the two other cohorts. At 8 years of survivorship, the components free of revision for any cause were 90.9% for the TM + SS cohort, 84.9% for the TM + LS group, and 90.6% for the NC + LS cohort (Fig. 13.2). The utilization of a short cemented tibial stem combined with a TM cone in rTKA offered identical survival rate with better functional result compared with the employment of a long uncemented stem associated with TM cones or metallic augments at a minimum of 5 years of follow-up [5].

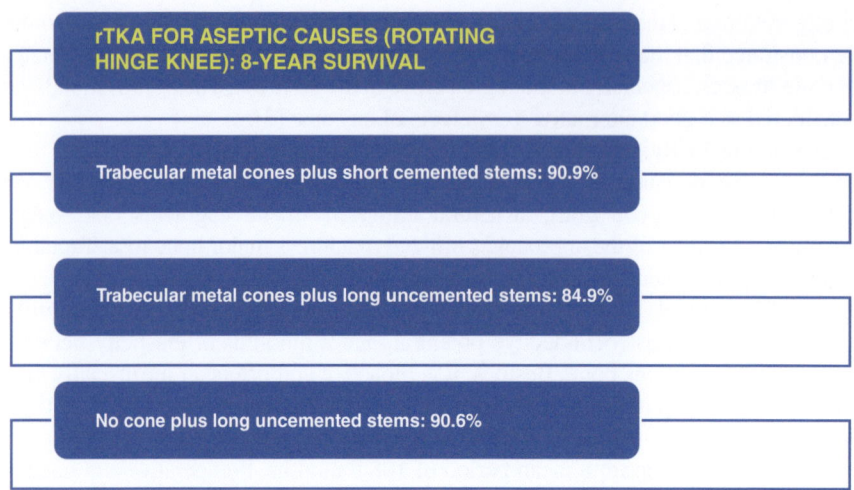

Fig. 13.2 Survivorship of revision total knee arthroplasty (rTKA) procedures for aseptic causes utilizing a rotating hinge knee at 8-year follow-up

In 2022, Spinello et al. described the surgical procedure and clinical and radiographic results of individuals treated with porous tantalum metaphyseal cones in combination with long uncemented diaphyseal-engaging stems to manage tibial bone loss in rTKA. Thirty-six aseptic rTKAs were carried out between 2016 and 2019. A single trabecular metal tantalum cone combined with a long (100 or 155 mm) press-fit, diaphyseal-engaging stem was utilized in all cases to reconstruct metaphyseal osseous defects and to augment tibial fixation. Cemented stems were excluded. The mean KSS and Knee Society Function Score (KSS-F) improved substantially from 29.7 points preoperatively to 86 points and from 20.4 points preoperatively to 72.3 points, respectively. Eleven tibial constructs (30.5%) had incomplete, nonprogressive radiolucent lines (≤2 mm). All tibial cones showed osteointegration. One individual experienced a full revision for periprosthetic joint infection (PJI), and survivorship free of any component revision was 91.7% at final follow-up. Hybrid fixation with uncemented diaphyseal-engaging stems and porous tantalum metaphyseal cones resulted in radiographic lack of osteolysis, good clinical results, and survivorship of 91.7% at a median follow-up of 33 months when considering all-cause revision as the endpoint [6].

13.3 Polyethylene (PE) Thickness

In a study with level 4 of evidence published in 2020 by Lo Presti et al., it was stated that bone defects during revision procedures for failed unicompartmental knee arthroplasty (UKA) represent a challenge even for the most expert orthopedic surgeons; consequently, a precise preoperative planning endures crucial to avert dramatic scenarios in the surgical theatre. Lo Presti et al. thought that bearing thickness utilized in original UKA represented a dependable predictor of severe tibial bone loss, needing a metallic augment or constrained implant, during revision to TKA. Forty-two patients who underwent a TKA from failed UKA were assessed clinically utilizing the KSS. A posterior-stabilized (PS) prosthesis was utilized in 27 cases (64.3%). An augment was needed in 12 individuals (28.6%). Initial bearing thickness greater than 8 mm was related to greater probability of a varus-valgus constrained (VVC) implant and a tibial augment. Tibial tray design, patients' gender or age during revision surgery, and side or cause of failure were not related to increased risk of augmentation or constrained implants [7].

13.4 Stem Length

According to Patel et al. (2015), biomechanical studies have demonstrated that TKA stems increase the mechanical stability by transferring load over a larger area and therefore diminish strain at the bone-component interface. The length of a rTKA stem is determined by the patient's anatomy and the intended fixation, namely, fully cemented or press-fit cortical contact. The pros and cons of various stem lengths must be weighed against the needs of the individual to accomplish an optimal result [8].

In 2017, Fleischman et al. stated that although the need for stemmed components was well accepted to improve mechanical survival in rTKA, the ideal fixation method and stem design endured dubious. They carried out a retrospective review of 223 individuals who experienced rTKA in whom stemmed components had not been utilized previously and with a mean follow-up of 61.6 months, including 108 components with fully cemented stems and 316 components with "hybrid" press-fit stems. They found that the risk for mechanical failure was equivalent for both cemented and hybrid stems. Young age was the single greatest risk factor for mechanical failure. Intramedullary canal fill, not stem length or diameter, was the strongest predictor of failure with hybrid stems, and risk was diminished by 41.2% for each additional 10% canal fill. In conclusion, both cemented and hybrid modular stems were viable alternatives in rTKA. Orthopedic surgeons should try to maximize canal filling of hybrid stems to get a solid press fit [9].

In 2018, Ettinger et al. affirmed that hyperextension of the femoral component and excessive slope of the tibial component might delay the cam-post engagement in semi-constrained rTKA. Further, it may compromise the posterior condylar offset (PCO). They stated that no previous study has determined whether a short 50-mm stem or longer stems (100 mm and 150 mm) resulted in less hyperextension of the femoral component or excessive slope and its impact on the PCO. Flexion/extension of the femoral component with respect to the sagittal femoral anatomic axis of the distal diaphysis (SFAA) and the tibial slope were measured from rotationally controlled lateral X-rays of 126 individuals with a one- or two-stage rTKA. Stems of 50 mm, 100 mm, and 150 mm were analyzed. They found that because 50-mm stems resulted in about three-degree hyperextension of the femoral component with respect to the SFAA compared to 100-mm or 150-mm stems, the longer stems do not modify the natural femoral flexion and a delay of the cam-post engagement may be averted. Further, a better reconstruction of the PCO might be accomplished with the utilization of longer stems [10].

Kang et al. (2018) stated that although stems improved initial mechanical stability in rTKA, ideal indications, proper lengths and diameters, and appropriate fixation techniques endured dubious. They affirmed that the stem length and diameter should be tailored according to patients' anatomical characteristics and determined fixation strategy. There were two methods of stem fixation including the total cementation technique and the hybrid technique with a cementless press-fit stem. Selection of a cementation technique should be based on exhaustive consideration of pros and cons of each method [11].

13.5 Tibial Baseplate

According to MacDonald and Vasarhelyi (2017), tibial baseplate roughness and PE-insert micromotion due to locking-mechanism loosening can result in PE backside wear in TKAs. They analyzed six tibial inserts retrieved at the time of TKA. The study demonstrated that in the complex interplay between baseplate surface finish and locking mechanism design, a polished baseplate with a robust locking mechanism had the lowest backside damage and linear wear [12].

In a study with level 3 of evidence published in 2020 by Robertsson et al., they affirmed that modern modular implants permit orthopedic surgeons to mix different combinations of components within the same brand. In this Swedish registry study, they found a higher loosening risk with the pegged baseplate than the stemmed one, even after controlling for age and sex [13].

King et al. (2022) analyzed the outcomes of pTKA in the morbidly obese (body mass index, BMI ≥ 40) patient utilizing a highly porous cementless tibial baseplate. This was a retrospective study of 167 primary TKAs (pTKAs) in individuals with morbid obesity experiencing primary cementless TKA with a minimum 5-year follow-up. Six individuals died and 14 were lost to follow-up, leaving 147 pTKAs in 136 individuals with a mean follow-up of 66 months. The average age was 59 years and average BMI was 45 kg/m^2. Clinical outcomes, patient-reported outcome measures (PROMS), radiographs, and adverse events were reviewed. There were nine failures needing revision, including three for aseptic tibial loosening (2%), two for deep infection (1.4%), two for patellar resurfacing (1.4%), one for patella instability (0.7%), and one for extensor mechanism rupture (0.7%). KSS improved from 48 to 90 at 2- and 5-year follow-up. KSS function score improved from 49 to 68 and 79 at 2- and 5-year follow-up, respectively. Survivorship with aseptic loosening as the endpoint was 98% at 5 years. Cementless TKA utilizing a highly porous tibial baseplate in morbidly obese individuals showed excellent clinical outcomes with 98% survivorship at 5 years and seemed to offer durable long-run biologic fixation as an alternative to mechanical cement fixation in this challenging group of individuals [14].

Stevenson et al. (2022) stated that tibial component aseptic loosening endured problematic in pTKA. Influential factors include component design, metallurgy, and cement method. Besides, reports advised for longer tibial stem fixation in high BMI individuals. They used a single stem length modular titanium baseplate in individuals regardless of BMI, bone quality, or malalignment. This design of a specific modular titanium base plate with a cruciate-shaped keel and grit blast surface showed 99% survivorship regardless of individual BMI or malalignment over 7-year follow-up period. Consistent cement technique with high viscosity cement indicated that component design endured an important variable impacting survivorship in pTKA [15].

According to Cooperman et al. (2022), a common tibial construct for rTKA includes a long diaphyseal engaging press-fit stem. Due to tibial canal bowing, compromises are frequently needed to match patient anatomy when choosing stemmed implants. They investigated through 3-D modeling whether implant press-fit alternatives adequately fit patient anatomy or whether an alternative angle between the stem and baseplate could increase the cortical engagement of long press-fit tibial stems. They found that custom free-angle stem placement permitted for increased stem diameter and cortical contact of press-fit tibial stems compared to existing constructs that must interface with the baseplate at a 90-degree angle [16].

In 2023, Awwad et al. affirmed that with the growing demand for TKA in a younger cohort of individuals, there has been an increasing interest in cementless tibial baseplate fixation. They analyzed whether there was a clear advantage to the utilization of three different forms of tibial baseplate fixation. The primary outcome of this study was survivorship and secondary outcomes were functional and radiological outcomes, up until 10 years. Awwad et al. performed a randomized controlled trial and recruited 224 individuals with 274 knees. Individuals experienced TKA by a single surgeon using a standard surgical technique. All individuals received a cruciate retaining TKA with a cementless femoral component and were randomized to receive either a cemented tibial component, a pegged porous coated cementless tibial component with screws, or a cementless tantalum monoblock tibial component with pegs. PROMS, radiological data, and survivorship were evaluated until 10 years postoperatively. Preoperative ROM, alignment, and PROMS were similar between the three cohorts. The utilization of cemented, cementless with screws, or cementless with pegs fixation options leads to differences in functional results. There was greater improvement in the Oxford score and KSS in individuals who received a cemented baseplate compared to tantalum and the pegged porous cohorts. However, radiological and survival results were similar in all three cohorts. Overall survivorship was 99.6%, with one knee with cementless tibial fixation and screws revised for subsidence at 3 years. There were no cases of venous thromboembolism, periprosthetic fracture, or infection. Irrespective of tibial fixation method, functional and radiological results remained similar at follow-up at 10 years, with no clear difference in result between each cohort. Each technique of fixation also had excellent survivorship over this period and should reassure orthopedic surgeons that whichever method of fixation they choose, long-run results are likely to be satisfactory [17].

13.6 Conclusions

In complex pTKAs and rTKAs (severe femoral and tibial metaphyseal bone defects), very good mid-run survivorship of tantalum metal cones has been reported. The utilization of a short cemented tibial stem combined with a trabecular metal (TM) cone in rTKA offers identical survival rate compared with the employment of a long uncemented stem associated with TM cones or metallic augments at a minimum of 5 years of follow-up. Hybrid fixation with uncemented diaphyseal-engaging stems and porous tantalum metaphyseal cones results in survivorship of 91.7% at a median follow-up of 33 months when considering all-cause revision as the endpoint. Initial bearing thickness greater than 8 mm is related to greater probability of a VVC implant and a tibial augment. Both cemented and hybrid modular stems are viable alternatives in rTKA. Orthopedic surgeons should try to maximize canal filling of hybrid stems to get a solid press fit. A polished baseplate with a robust locking mechanism has the lowest backside damage and linear wear. Custom free-angle stem placement permits for increased stem diameter and cortical contact of press-fit tibial stems compared to existing constructs that must interface with the baseplate at a 90-degree angle. Cemented tibial component, a pegged porous coated cementless tibial component with screws, or a cementless tantalum monoblock tibial component with pegs give similar results at follow-up at 10 years.

References

1. LaMonica J, Pham N, Milligan K, Tommasini SM, Schwarzkopf R, Parisi R, et al. How metal augments, polyethylene thickness and stem length affect tibial baseplate load transfer in revision total knee arthroplasty. Knee. 2023;40:283–91. https://doi.org/10.1016/j.knee.2022.11.021.
2. Sculco PK, Abdel MP, Hanssen AD, Lewallen DG. The management of bone loss in revision total knee arthroplasty: rebuild, reinforce, and augment. Bone Joint J. 2016;98-B(1 Suppl A):120–4. https://doi.org/10.1302/0301-620X.98B1.36345.
3. Innocenti B, Fekete G, Pianigiani S. Biomechanical analysis of augments in revision total knee arthroplasty. J Biomech Eng. 2018;140(11):111006. https://doi.org/10.1115/1.4040966.
4. Rajgopal A, Kumar S, Aggarwal K. Midterm outcomes of tantalum metal cones for severe bone loss in complex primary and revision total knee arthroplasty. Arthroplast Today. 2021;7:76–83. https://doi.org/10.1016/j.artd.2020.12.004.
5. Jacquet C, Ros F, Guy S, Parratte S, Ollivier M, Argenson JN. Trabecular metal cones combined with short cemented stem allow favorable outcomes in aseptic revision total knee arthroplasty. J Arthroplasty. 2021;36(2):657–63. https://doi.org/10.1016/j.arth.2020.08.058.
6. Spinello P, Thiele RAR, Zepeda K, Giori N, Indelli PF. The use of tantalum cones and diaphyseal-engaging stems in tibial component revision: a consecutive series. Knee Surg Relat Res. 2022;34(1):12. https://doi.org/10.1186/s43019-022-00141-7.
7. Lo Presti M, Costa GG, Grassi A, Agrò G, Cialdella S, Vasco C, et al. Bearing thickness of unicompartmental knee arthroplasty is a reliable predictor of tibial bone loss during revision to total knee arthroplasty. Orthop Traumatol Surg Res. 2020;106(3):429–34. https://doi.org/10.1016/j.otsr.2019.12.018.
8. Patel AR, Barlow B, Ranawat AS. Stem length in revision total knee arthroplasty. Curr Rev Musculoskelet Med. 2015;8(4):407–12. https://doi.org/10.1007/s12178-015-9297-4.

9. Fleischman AN, Azboy I, Fuery M, Restrepo C, Shao H, Parvizi J. Effect of stem size and fixation method on mechanical failure after revision total knee arthroplasty. J Arthroplasty. 2017;32(9S):S202–S208.e1. https://doi.org/10.1016/j.arth.2017.04.055.
10. Ettinger M, Savov P, Balubaid O, Windhagen H, Calliess T. Influence of stem length on component flexion and posterior condylar offset in revision total knee arthroplasty. Knee. 2018;25(3):480–4. https://doi.org/10.1016/j.knee.2018.02.011.
11. Kang SG, Park CH, Song SJ. Stem fixation in revision total knee arthroplasty: indications, stem dimensions, and fixation methods. Knee Surg Relat Res. 2018;30(3):187–92. https://doi.org/10.5792/ksrr.18.019.
12. Sisko ZW, Teeter MG, Lanting BA, Howard JL, McCalden RW, Naudie DD, et al. Current total knee designs: does baseplate roughness or locking mechanism design affect polyethylene backside wear? Clin Orthop Relat Res. 2017;475(12):2970–80. https://doi.org/10.1007/s11999-017-5494-3.
13. Robertsson O, Sundberg M, Sezgin EA, Lidgren L, W-Dahl A. Higher risk of loosening for a four-pegged TKA tibial baseplate than for a stemmed one: a register-based study. Clin Orthop Relat Res. 2020;478(1):58–65. https://doi.org/10.1097/CORR.0000000000000774.
14. King BA, Miller AJ, Nadar AC, Smith LS, Yakkanti MR, Harwin SF, et al. Cementless total knee arthroplasty using a highly porous tibial baseplate in morbidly obese patients: minimum 5-year follow-up. J Knee Surg. 2023;36(9):995–1000. https://doi.org/10.1055/s-0042-1748900.
15. Stevenson KL, Blackburn BE, Da Silva AZ, Erickson JA, Anderson LA, Pelt CE, et al. High survivorship of a modular titanium baseplate independent of body mass index and malalignment. J Arthroplasty. 2022;37(6S):S216–20. https://doi.org/10.1016/j.arth.2022.02.006.
16. Cooperman C, Wiznia D, Kunsel K, Roytman G, Ani L, Pratola D, et al. Personalizing revision tibial baseplate position and stem trajectory with custom implants using 3D modeling to optimize press-fit stem placement. Arthroplast Today. 2022;18:45–51. https://doi.org/10.1016/j.artd.2022.08.011.
17. Awwad GEH, Ahedi H, Angadi D, Kandhari V, Coolican MRJ. A prospective randomised controlled trial of cemented and uncemented tibial baseplates: functional and radiological outcomes. Arch Orthop Trauma Surg. 2023;143(9):5891–9. https://doi.org/10.1007/s00402-023-04831-z.

Cementless Porous-Coated Metaphyseal Sleeves Used for Bone Defects in Revision Total Knee Arthroplasty

14

E. Carlos Rodríguez-Merchán, Carlos A. Encinas-Ullán, Juan S. Ruiz-Pérez, and Primitivo Gómez-Cardero

14.1 Introduction

According to Mancuso et al. (2017), revision total knee arthroplasty (rTKA) is commonly made more complex by the presence of bone defects, which might be caused by periprosthetic joint infection (PJI), polyethylene (PE) wear, implant loosening, or fractures. In a literature review, they found that Anderson Orthopaedic Research Institute (AORI) classification was the most commonly utilized because it helped in the choice of the most suitable management (Fig. 14.1). Several alternatives were available in the treatment of metaphyseal bone loss in rTKA. For small and contained defects (AORI type 1), cement with or without screws and auto- or allograft morselized bone were available. In uncontained but mild defects (AORI type 2A), metal augments should be utilized, while large and uncontained defects (AORI type 2B and 3) were best addressed with structural allograft or metal filling devices (cones and sleeves). Stemmed components, either cemented or cementless, were advised to diminish the strain at the implant-host interface. The conclusion of this publication was that management of bone defects in rTKA had evolved during the last years providing different alternatives with good outcomes at a short-/medium-run follow-up. Long-run clinical result and implant survival following rTKA were still suboptimal and depended upon many factors including cause for revision, surgical approach, type of implants utilized, and various patient factors [1].

The purpose of this chapter is to review recent advances on cementless porous-coated metaphyseal sleeves used for bone defects in rTKA.

E. C. Rodríguez-Merchán (✉) · C. A. Encinas-Ullán · J. S. Ruiz-Pérez · P. Gómez-Cardero
Department of Orthopedic Surgery, La Paz University Hospital, Madrid, Spain

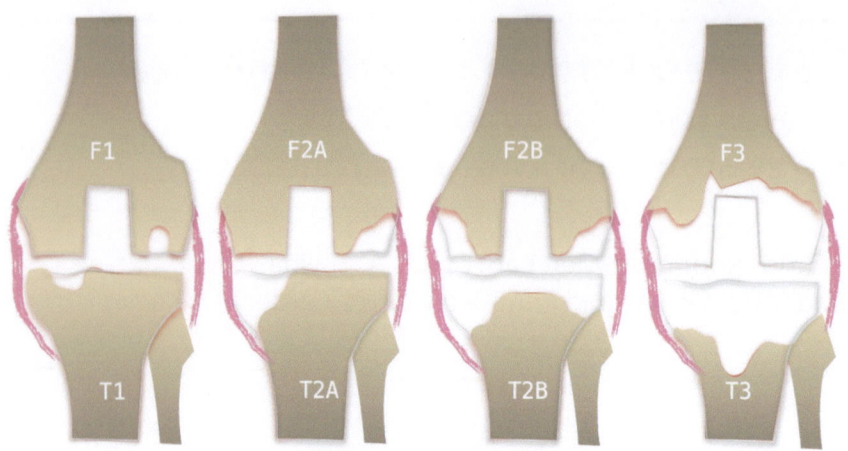

Fig. 14.1 Anderson Orthopaedic Research Institute (AORI) radiographic classification system for bone loss in patients undergoing revision total knee arthroplasty (rTKA)

14.2 Indications and Contraindications

According to Graichen et al., the indications of cementless metaphyseal sleeves are all tibial and femoral osseous defects AORI grade 2 and 3. The contraindications are cases where stable uncemented fixation of the metaphyseal implant is not feasible [2].

If after the removal of the femoral component the distal femur has poor bone stock, it is important not to downsize the femur to match the remaining bone; in addition, we cannot rely on lots of cement to fill all these zones of missing bone; in this circumstance, metal augment (blocks) can be used to fill the gaps of missing bone; when the bone loss is too great, augments cannot be utilized; on the contrary, a cone or sleeve must be used use to bypass the distal femur and engage bone more proximal either the metaphysis or diaphysis (Fig. 14.2).

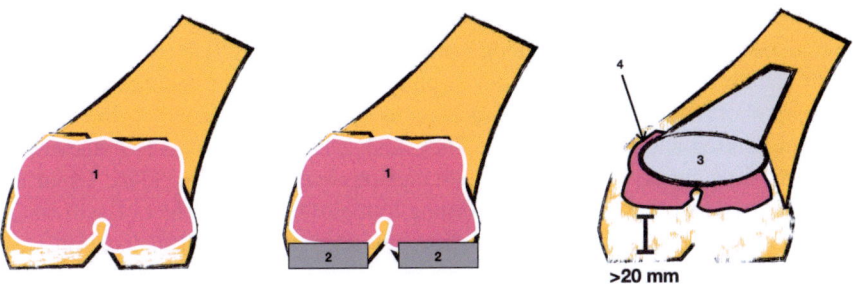

Fig. 14.2 Distal femur following removal of femoral implant (poor bone stock): We don't desire to downsize the femur to match the remaining bone, but we cannot rely on a great quantity of cement to fill all the areas of missing bone (**left**); we can use metal augment (blocks) to fill the gaps of the missing bone (**center**); when the bone loss is too great, we cannot utilize augments; we must then use a cone or sleeve to bypass the distal femur and engage bone more proximal either the metaphysis or diaphysis (**right**). 1 = remaining bone; 2 = metal augments; 3 = metal sleeve; 4 = little remaining bone

14.3 Results

Between 2007 and 2011, 193 sleeves (119 tibial/74 femoral) were implanted in 121 aseptic rTKAs by Graichen et al. (2015). After the average of 3.6 years, they were analyzed clinically and radiographically. The AKSS (American Knee Society Score) increased from 88 to 147 points. Range of motion (ROM) increased from 89 to 114. Overall revision rate was 11.6%. Four sleeves were revised for aseptic loosening (2% of total sleeves). Ten revisions were carried out mainly for infection (3.3%) or ligament instability (3.3%) [2].

In 2017, Watters et al. assessed the mid-run outcomes of stepped, porous-coated metaphyseal sleeves in rTKA in the setting of severe osseous loss. Individuals who experienced rTKA utilizing metaphyseal sleeves from March 2006 to May 2014 were analyzed. Preoperative patient characteristics and operative information were reviewed. Postoperative results were compared with preoperative values. Primary study outcomes included adverse events, reoperations, radiographic evaluation of sleeve osteointegration, and survivorship. One hundred sixteen knees (108 individuals) experienced rTKA with 152 metaphyseal sleeves (111 tibial and 41 femoral). AORI defect classification included five type 2A, 89 type 2B, and 17 type 3 tibial defects and three type 2A, 34 type 2B, and four type 3 femoral defects. Three intraoperative fractures (1.9%) associated with sleeve preparation and/or insertion occurred. Six knees (five individuals) were lost to follow-up and five individuals (six knees) died before 2 years. Of the remaining 104 knees (98 individuals, 134 sleeves), mean follow-up was 5.3 years. Nineteen knees (16.4%) needed reoperation, most frequently for recurrent infection. Only one sleeve showed radiographic evidence of failed osteointegration but did not need revision. Two sleeves (1.5%) needed removal and/or resection for recurrent infection. This study illustrated the utility of porous metaphyseal sleeves in rTKA with a low percentage of intraoperative adverse events, excellent osteointegration, and long-run fixation [3].

In a study with level 4 of evidence published in 2018 by Fedorka et al., they assessed short-run outcomes of porous-coated metaphyseal sleeves with regard to implant fixation and clinical results. They analyzed 50 individuals (79 sleeves: 49 tibial and 30 femoral) who had a press-fit metaphyseal sleeve with rTKA. Tibial and femoral bone loss was classified according to the AORI bone defect classification. Postoperative adverse events of infection, revision surgery, and dislocation were evaluated. Follow-up radiographs were assessed for signs of loosening utilizing the criteria developed by the Knee Society. The median follow-up was 58.8 months. The bone loss classifications were one type 1, 30 type 2A, two type 2B, and 17 type 3, and with regard to the femur, five were type 1, eight type 2A, 31 type 2B, and six type 3. At final follow-up, 41/45 (91.1%) tibial and 28/29 (96.6%) femoral sleeves demonstrated radiographic evidence of ingrowth. Of these 69 individuals, all exhibited radiographic evidence of bony ingrowth. Three sleeves were revised for infection and two for loosening. The reoperation percentage for loosening was 6.8% (5/74) and for any reason was 18.9% (14/74). Modular porous-coated press-fit metaphyseal sleeves filled defects and provided evidence of radiographic ingrowth. The conclusion of this study was that short-run stable fixation can be accomplished with sleeves, which is helpful as more individuals experience rTKA with greater bone loss [4].

In a systematic review of the literature published in 2018 by Zanirato et al., they summarized indications, adverse events, and clinical and radiological mid-run outcomes of metaphyseal sleeves in the treatment of bone defects in rTKA. Retrospective or prospective studies with 2 years of follow-up were included. Thirteen articles with a level of evidence of IV were included. One thousand seventy-nine rTKAs (1554 sleeves) with a mean follow-up of 4 years were analyzed. The studies demonstrated good clinical and functional results. Sleeves permitted a stable metaphyseal fixation and osteointegration with an implant and sleeves' aseptic survival percentage of 97.7% and 99.2%, respectively. The prevalence of PJI was 2.7%. The estimated percentage of reoperations and re-revisions were 14.2% and 7.1%, respectively. Metaphyseal sleeves represented a viable alternative in treatment of types 2b and 3 AORI bone defects in rTKA [5].

In a study with level 3 of evidence published in 2020 by Klim et al., they analyzed the implant durability and the clinical and the radiological mid-run outcomes in rTKA when utilizing metaphyseal sleeves. Clinical and radiological follow-up examinations were carried out in 92 individuals (93 knees) with rTKA utilizing hybrid fixation method (cementless sleeves and stem). Radiographic measurements regarding osteointegration at the sleeve-bone interface were carried out, and the ROM, a subjective satisfaction score (SSS), the American Knee Society Score (KSS), the Western Ontario and McMaster Universities Osteoarthritis Index (WOMAC), as well as the SF-36 Health survey were examined. Bone defects were analyzed utilizing the AORI classification. No knee had to be revised due to aseptic loosening at the time of the follow-up (mean 6.3 years, minimum 2 years). Satisfactory radiographic osteointegration at the sleeve-bone interface was found in 96.1% of cases. Seventeen knees (18.2%) had to be re-revised, 15 of them due to a recurrent infection and two due to aseptic reasons (mediolateral instability and a periprosthetic fracture). The median of the ROM (96°), SSS (8), KSS (87), WOMAC (9), SF-36 mental component summary (55), and SF-36 physical component summary (38) demonstrated very satisfying outcomes. No case of aseptic loosening was encountered in this series. This study showed that the utilization of metaphyseal sleeves is an excellent management alternative for extended bone defects in rTKA surgery [6].

In 2023, Shen et al. investigated clinical and radiographic mid-run results of the sleeves for the treatment of metaphyseal bone defects in rTKAs. From 2015 to 2019, 44 individuals (45 knees) who were operated with cementless porous-coated metaphyseal sleeve in rTKA were analyzed. Bone defects were evaluated according to AORI classification. On the tibial side, there were 37 type 2 and six type 3, and with regard to the femur, 15 were type 2, and four were type 3. Through reviewing electronic records, information was collected, including baseline demographics, operative details, information of prosthesis, and adverse events. Clinical and radiographic evaluations were performed, including KSS, WOMAC, ROM, the radiolucent line, level of joint line, and implant survival percentage. The mean follow-up time was 4.4 years. During surgery, sleeve-related fractures were found in four (8.9%) knees, including incomplete tibial fracture of the lateral cortex in one knee and of medial cortex in two knees and longitudinal femoral metaphyseal fracture in one knee. Unions were accomplished in all cases at the final follow-up. Substantial improvements in KSS and WOMAC scores were encountered at the final follow-up, respectively, from 83.8 to 152.9 and from 148.4 to 88.1. The mean ROM improved from 88.7° to 113.7°. A 75-mm length of cementless stem was utilized in all individuals, and only one individual was identified as tibial end-of-stem pain. No sleeve-related revision happened, and one individual was diagnosed with early postoperative infection and was treated with irrigation and debridement, PE liner exchange, and adequate antibiotic treatment. The overall implant survival was 97.8% with the endpoint reoperation and 100% with the endpoint revision. Osteointegration at the sleeve-bone interface was encountered in all individuals and no loosening occurred. Satisfactory alignment between 3° varus and 3° valgus was accomplished in all but not in three individuals. The utilization of metaphyseal sleeves in the management of bone defects in rTKAs can provide stable fixation and substantially improve the clinical scores at the mid-run follow-up. Besides, the rare occurrence of end-of-stem pain suggests routine utilization of cementless stems [7]. Figures 14.3 and 14.4 show two cases of aseptic loosening with large bone defect that required the use of metaphyseal sleeves to achieve a stable rTKA.

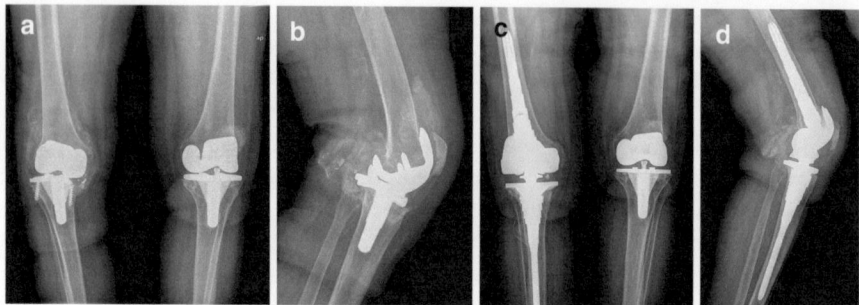

Fig. 14.3 (a–d) Aseptic loosening of a primary total knee arthroplasty (pTKA) of the right knee in a patient who had undergone bilateral pTKA. Preoperative anteroposterior (AP) (**a**) and lateral (**b**) radiographs of the right knee showed a significant bony defect. Metaphyseal sleeves were used to achieve stability of the revision total knee arthroplasty (rTKA): postoperative AP radiograph (**c**); postoperative lateral radiograph (**d**)

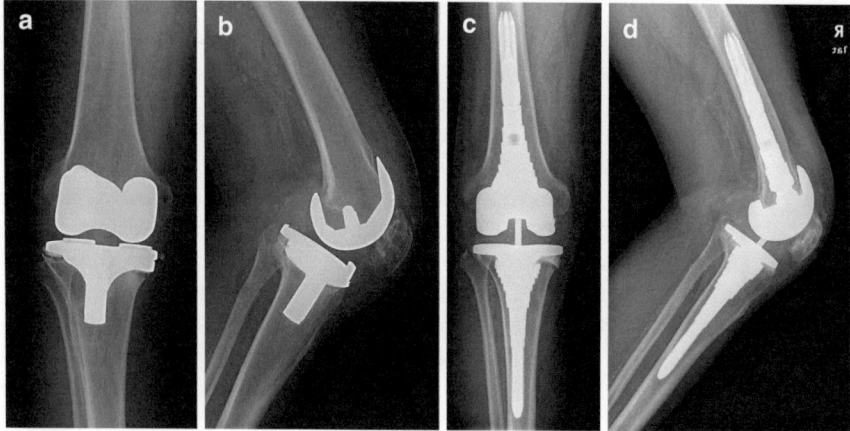

Fig. 14.4 (a–d) Aseptic loosening of a primary total knee arthroplasty (pTKA) of a patient's right knee. Preoperative anteroposterior (AP) (**a**) and lateral (**b**) radiographic images of the right knee showed a significant bony defect. Metaphyseal sleeves were used to achieve the stability of revision total knee arthroplasty (rTKA): postoperative AP radiograph (**c**); postoperative lateral radiograph (**d**)

14.4 Survivorship

In 2017, Chalmers et al. analyzed adverse events, re-revisions, and survivorship free of revision for aseptic loosening of metaphyseal sleeves in rTKA. Two hundred eighty individuals with 393 metaphyseal sleeves (144 femoral, 249 tibial) implanted during rTKA from 2006 to 2014 were analyzed. Sleeves were most frequently cemented (55% femoral, 72% tibial). Mean follow-up was 3 years, mean age was 66 years, and mean body mass index was 34 kg/m². Indications for rTKA included two-stage reimplantation for deep infection (37%), aseptic loosening of the tibia (14%), femur (12%), or both components (9%), and instability (14%). There was a 12% rate of perioperative adverse events, most frequently intraoperative fracture (6.5%). Eight sleeves (2.5%) required removal: 6 (2%) during component resection for deep infection (all were well fixed at removal) as well as 1 (0.8%) femoral sleeve and 1 (0.8%) tibial sleeve for aseptic loosening. Five-year survivorship free of revision for aseptic loosening was 96% and 99.5% for femoral and tibial sleeves, respectively. Level of constraint, bone loss, sleeve and/or stem fixation, and revision indication did not substantially influenced results. Metaphyseal sleeve fixation to enhance component stability during rTKA had a 5-year survivorship free of revision for aseptic loosening of 96% and 99.5% in femoral and tibial sleeves, respectively. Both cemented and cementless sleeve fixation provided dependable durability at intermediate follow-up [8].

In 2021, Rodríguez-Merchán et al. stated that higher-quality long-run studies should be performed to be able to reach scientifically firm conclusions about the true value of highly porous metal sleeves [9].

14.5 Conclusions

In a study, after average of 3.6 years, the overall revision rate was 11.6%. After a mean follow-up of 5.3 years, other authors had 1.9% intraoperative fractures associated with sleeve preparation and/or insertion: 16.4% needed reoperation, most frequently for recurrent infection. Only one sleeve showed radiographic evidence of failed osteointegration but did not need revision; 1.5% needed removal and/or resection for recurrent infection. In another report with a mean follow-up of 4.9 years, the reoperation percentage for loosening was 6.8% and for any reason was 18.9%. A systematic review with a mean follow-up of 4 years found that the implant and sleeves' aseptic survival rates were 97.7% and 99.2%, respectively. The prevalence of PJI was 2.7%. The estimated percentage of reoperations and re-revisions were 14.2% and 7.1%, respectively. Other reports with a mean follow-up of 6.3 years (minimum 2 years) found satisfactory radiographic osseointegration at the sleeve-bone interface in 96.1% of cases. The rate of re-revision was 18.2%. After a mean follow-up time of 4.4 years, other authors found an 8.9% of sleeve-related fractures during surgery. The overall implant survival was 97.8% with the endpoint reoperation and 100% with the endpoint revision. In another study, after a mean follow-up of 3 years, there was a 12% rate of perioperative adverse events, most frequently intraoperative fracture (6.5%). Five-year survivorship free of revision for aseptic loosening was 96% and 99.5% for femoral and tibial sleeves, respectively.

References

1. Mancuso F, Beltrame A, Colombo E, Miani E, Bassini F. Management of metaphyseal bone loss in revision knee arthroplasty. Acta Biomed. 2017;88(2S):98–111. https://doi.org/10.23750/abm.v88i2-S.6520.
2. Graichen H, Strauch M, Scior W, Morgan-Jones R. Knee revision arthroplasty: cementless, metaphyseal fixation with sleeves. Oper Orthop Traumatol. 2015;27(1):24–34. https://doi.org/10.1007/s00064-014-0333-0.
3. Watters TS, Martin JR, Levy DL, Yang CC, Kim RH, Dennis DA. Porous-coated metaphyseal sleeves for severe femoral and tibial bone loss in revision TKA. J Arthroplasty. 2017;32(11):3468–73. https://doi.org/10.1016/j.arth.2017.06.025.
4. Fedorka CJ, Chen AF, Pagnotto MR, Crossett LS, Klatt BA. Revision total knee arthroplasty with porous-coated metaphyseal sleeves provides radiographic ingrowth and stable fixation. Knee Surg Sports Traumatol Arthrosc. 2018;26(5):1500–5. https://doi.org/10.1007/s00167-017-4493-y.
5. Zanirato A, Cavagnaro L, Basso M, Divano S, Felli L, Formica M. Metaphyseal sleeves in total knee arthroplasty revision: complications, clinical and radiological results. A systematic review of the literature. Arch Orthop Trauma Surg. 2018;138(7):993–1001. https://doi.org/10.1007/s00402-018-2967-0.
6. Klim SM, Amerstorfer F, Bernhardt GA, Sadoghi P, Hauer G, Leitner L, et al. Excellent mid-term osseointegration and implant survival using metaphyseal sleeves in revision total knee arthroplasty. Knee Surg Sports Traumatol Arthrosc. 2020;28(12):3843–8. https://doi.org/10.1007/s00167-020-05865-1.
7. Shen J, Zhang T, Zhang Y, Dong Y, Zhou Y, Guo L. Cementless porous-coated metaphyseal sleeves used for bone defects in revision total knee arthroplasty: short- to mid-term outcomes. Orthop Surg. 2023;15(2):488–95. https://doi.org/10.1111/os.13598.
8. Chalmers BP, Desy NM, Pagnano MW, Trousdale RT, Taunton MJ. Survivorship of metaphyseal sleeves in revision total knee arthroplasty. J Arthroplasty. 2017;32(5):1565–70. https://doi.org/10.1016/j.arth.2016.12.004.
9. Rodríguez-Merchán EC, Gómez-Cardero P, Encinas-Ullán CA. Management of bone loss in revision total knee arthroplasty: therapeutic options and results. EFORT Open Rev. 2021;6(11):1073–86. https://doi.org/10.1302/2058-5241.6.210007.

Chronic Extensor Mechanism Failure After Primary or Revision Total Knee Arthroplasty: Reconstructive and Augmentation Options

15

E. Carlos Rodríguez-Merchán, Carlos A. Encinas-Ullán, Juan S. Ruiz-Pérez, and Primitivo Gómez-Cardero

15.1 Introduction

Extensor mechanism failure is a rare but severe adverse event after primary total knee arthroplasty (pTKA) or revision total knee arthroplasty (rTKA). It is associated with substantial morbidity and diminished quality of life due to extensor lag, instability, difficulty walking, and/or pain. Its prevalence is reported to be between 0.1% and 2.5% in all TKA, but rTKA is considered to carry a higher risk [1–5]. Primary repair of the chronic extensor mechanism failure has a very high failure percentage with unsatisfactory result and has consequently been abandoned [2, 6, 7]. Reconstructive and augmentation alternatives comprise autograft, allograft, synthetic graft, and medial gastrocnemius flap [2, 3, 5].

The purpose of this chapter is to review recent developments on reconstructive and augmentation options for chronic extensor mechanism failure after pTKA or rTKA.

15.2 Autograft

The semitendinosus tendon is the most frequently utilized autograft for reconstruction of chronic extensor mechanism disruption [2, 8]. The semitendinosus autograft was first described by Cadambi and Engh [8–10]. If additional augmentation is needed, a gracilis tendon can be utilized. However, the semitendinosus graft can only be utilized if the patella is not substantially retracted, and there is good bone quality remaining in the patella [2, 3].

In 2022, Masouros et al. reported on four individuals with chronic (>3 months) patellar tendon rupture after pTKA, who were treated with a new technique of

E. C. Rodríguez-Merchán (✉) · C. A. Encinas-Ullán · J. S. Ruiz-Pérez · P. Gómez-Cardero
Department of Orthopedic Surgery, La Paz University Hospital, Madrid, Spain

© The Author(s), under exclusive license to Springer Nature Switzerland AG 2024
E. C. Rodríguez-Merchán (ed.), *Advances in Revision Total Knee Arthroplasty*,
https://doi.org/10.1007/978-3-031-60445-4_15

staged patella advancement before reconstruction with autografts. Firstly, a unilateral frame was applied connecting the patella with the tibial shaft. The construct permitted for gradual distal advancement of the patella based on the Ilizarov principles. After accomplishing the desired patellar height, the frame was removed, and the patellar tendon was reconstructed with hamstrings. All four individuals experienced a substantial improvement in extensor lag by a mean of 38°, while Knee Society Scores (KSS) increased by a mean of 38.5 points. No significant loss in active knee flexion was encountered. The stage technique yielded favorable results [11].

15.3 Allograft

In the study of Emerson et al. published in 1990, 13 knees in 12 individuals were reconstructed utilizing an allograft distal extensor mechanism. The graft consisted of a quadriceps tendon, a patella with a cemented prosthesis, a patellar tendon, and a tibial tubercle. Knee extension power and improved function were obtained in all cases, although minimal extensor lags were present in three cases. Preoperative motion returned in all but one knee. Two graft adverse events happened, both in the first three after surgery: one quadriceps junction treated by re-suture failed at the 1-month mark, and the other graft had to be revised for extensor weakness from rupture of the graft at the patella-patellar tendon junction, which was attributed to surgical damage to the tendon. One individual fractured the allograft patella in a serious fall [12].

In 2005, Burnett et al. evaluated two techniques of reconstructing a disrupted extensor mechanism with the utilization of an extensor mechanism allograft in rTKA. Twenty reconstructions with the utilization of an extensor mechanism allograft consisting of the tibial tubercle, patellar tendon, patella, and quadriceps tendon were carried out. The first seven reconstructions (group I) were performed with the allograft minimally tensioned. The 13 subsequent procedures (group II) were done with the allograft tightly tensioned in full extension. All surviving allografts were assessed clinically and radiographically after a minimum duration of follow-up of 24 months. All of the reconstructions in group I were clinical failures, with an average postoperative extensor lag of 59 degrees and an average postoperative Hospital for Special Surgery (HSS) knee score of 52 points. All 13 reconstructions in group II were clinical successes, with an average postoperative extensor lag of 4.3° and an average HSS knee score of 88 points. Postoperative flexion did not differ substantially between group I (average, 108°) and group II (average, 104°). The outcomes of reconstruction with an extensor mechanism allograft after TKA depended on the initial tensioning of the allograft. Loosely tensioned allografts led to a persistent extension lag and clinical failure. Allografts that are tightly tensioned in full extension can restore active knee extension and lead to clinical success [13]. Figure 15.1 shows a scheme of the surgical technique of extensor mechanism allograft. Figure 15.2 shows a case of severe chronic disruption of extensor mechanism treated by means of a complete patellar tendon allograft.

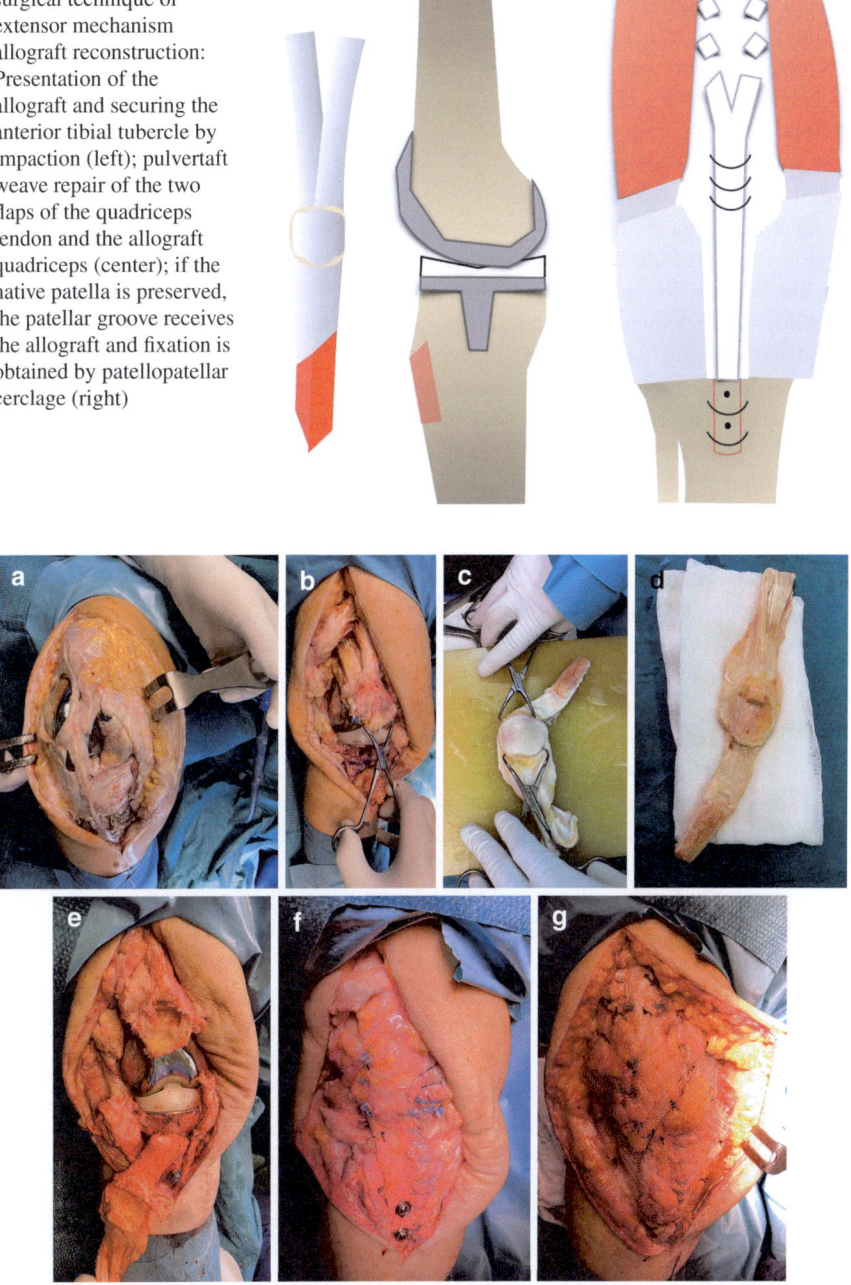

Fig. 15.1 Scheme of the surgical technique of extensor mechanism allograft reconstruction: Presentation of the allograft and securing the anterior tibial tubercle by impaction (left); pulvertaft weave repair of the two flaps of the quadriceps tendon and the allograft quadriceps (center); if the native patella is preserved, the patellar groove receives the allograft and fixation is obtained by patellopatellar cerclage (right)

Fig. 15.2 Severe chronic disruption of extensor mechanism (**a**); after debridement (**b**); complete patellar tendon allograft (**c**); definitive preparation of the graft and bone pad in tibial tubercle and patella (**d**); patella with "box" to accommodate the graft and distal fixation with two screws in the tibial tubercle (**e**); proximal reconstruction of patellar soft tissues with high-strength sutures (**f**); mesh augmentation (**g**)

In 2008, Malhotra et al. described a technique of extensor mechanism reconstruction for patellar tendon loss, after TKA, with the help of extensor mechanism composite allograft. Four individuals with chronic extensor mechanism-deficient TKA were undertaken for revision surgery along with reconstruction of extensor mechanism with a technique utilizing an extensor mechanism composite allograft consisting of a patella-patellar tendon-tibial tubercle. On final follow-up, none of the individuals had extensor lag but for 10° of extensor lag in one individual only [14].

Diaz-Ledesma et al. (2014) presented the outcomes of a protocol using Achilles tendon allograft followed by an abbreviated immobilization program to treat extensor mechanism disruptions after TKA in 29 knees (27 individuals). Failed reconstruction was defined as mechanical allograft failure needing re-intervention, extension lag >30°, recurrent falls, regression to a lower ambulatory status, and revision due to infection. With mean follow-up of 3.5 years, 17 cases (58.6%) had satisfactory outcomes, 11 cases (37.9%) were considered failures, and 1 case was lost to follow-up. Among failures, eight (27.5%) experienced reoperation with four (13.8%) due to late infections. This study suggested that a shortened immobilization protocol yields less favorable outcomes than expected and that continuous monitoring of individuals who had allograft reconstruction for possible development of late infection should be advised [15].

In a study with level 4 of evidence published in 2015 by Boettner and Bou Monsef, they described the surgical technique and early clinical outcomes of a modified Hanssen patelloplasty with an Achilles tendon allograft. The modified technique described in three individuals experiencing revision TKA aimed to augment the extensor mechanism by securing an Achilles tendon allograft to the proximal part of the patellar tendon and the distal quadriceps tendon utilizing mattress sutures. This served to reinforce the extensor mechanism and diminish the risk of a tear of its patellar attachment. The patellar bone defect was grafted using cortico-cancellous bone chips. Over a 12- to 48-month follow-up, all reconstructions healed with an increase in patellar bone thickness. No individual had any extensor lag, and all individuals accomplished 110°–125° of flexion. The Western Ontario and McMaster University Osteoarthritis Index knee scores improved from 53 preoperatively to 88.5 at last follow-up, with no reported adverse events. Augmentation of the extensor mechanism with an Achilles tendon permitted for early mobilization and excellent postoperative range of motion (ROM) in individuals with large patella bone defects and imminent patella fracture [16].

In 2017, Lim et al. presented the clinical and radiographic outcomes of reconstruction after extensor mechanism disruption in TKA individuals. Sixteen individuals with a mean age of 61 years at extensor mechanism reconstruction with a minimum of 2-year follow-up were included. The mean follow-up was 3.3 years. KSS before and at final follow-up extension lag, ROM, and radiographic change in patellar height were analyzed. There were statistically significant improvements between preoperative and final follow-up KSS for pain and function. The extension lag was also diminished from 35° preoperatively to 14° at final follow-up. There was an average proximal patellar migration of 8 mm. Five (31%) individuals had an extensor lag of >30° or revision surgery for repeat extensor mechanism reconstruction, infection, or arthrodesis. This 10-year experience utilizing allografts during extensor mechanism reconstruction showed reasonable results, but failures are to be forecast in about one-third of individuals [17].

In a study with level 4 of evidence published in 2022 by Helito et al., they reported the ROM, failure rate, and adverse events of individuals with extensor mechanism injury after TKA treated with extensor mechanism allograft with midrun follow-up. Individuals experiencing extensor mechanism transplantation from 2009 to 2018 were assessed. Demographics, the cause of transplantation, elapsed time from arthroplasty to transplantation, related surgical factors, immobilization time, ROM, transplant failure, and adverse events were collected. The minimum follow-up was 24 months. Twenty individuals were assessed. The mean follow-up was 70.8 months. The most frequent cause of extensor mechanism rupture was traumatic in 10 (50%) cases. Six individuals experienced associated surgeries, one case of medial ligament complex reconstruction, and five cases of rTKA. Eleven individuals (55%) had transplant-related adverse events. The most frequent adverse event was an infection. Five individuals presented transplant failure. Individuals who experienced extensor mechanism allograft transplantation after TKA had a 25% failure rate with a mean follow-up of 6 years [18].

15.4 Synthetic Graft

According to Abdel et al. (2019), Marlex mesh reconstruction of the extensor mechanism via a stepwise surgical approach is a viable alternative to manage disruption of the extensor mechanism after TKA. Extensor mechanism reconstruction with mesh involves a stepwise surgical approach with a particular monofilament polypropylene mesh (Marlex; C.R. Bard). The procedure averts the limitations of allograft with regard to availability, cost, and risk of illness transmission. The procedure is reproducible and cost-effective, and it has excellent functional and survivorship results [19].

In 2020, Giuntoli et al. reported their experience in the management of patellar tendon ruptures after TKA utilizing the Ligament Advanced Reinforcement System (LARS®). Clinical assessment was carried out utilizing the KSS and recording extensor lag. Instrumental assessment was carried out utilizing ultrasound imaging to evaluate patellar tendon thickness and utilizing conventional X-rays to evaluate prosthesis' mobilization signs and patellar height. At the final follow-up, six knees were included in their study. Patient's mean age was 66.7. Patellar tendon reconstruction happened after a mean time of 4 months from the previous surgery. The mean follow-up was 44.2 months. The mean knee score was 63.3 and the mean function score was 35. In four knees, the extensor lag was <10°, while in two knees, it was >20°. The mean Insall-Salvati Index was 1.16, while the average increment in tendon thickness was 127.12%. Giuntolli et al. thought that synthetic ligaments can be successfully used for the reconstruction of patellar tendon breakage after pTKA and rTKA in selected individuals [20].

In 2022, Fuchs et al. stated that lesions of the quadriceps or patellar tendon after total TKA were uncommon, but serious complications, if left untreated, can result in loss of function of the knee joint. They affirmed that chronic deficiencies are frequently related to multiple prior revision surgeries for joint infection or aseptic TKA failure, that biological allograft reconstruction showed unsatisfying outcomes, and that the use of a monofilament polypropylene mesh is a promising approach for this pathological condition. In their study, they assess clinical, functional, and patient-reported outcomes (PROMS) of this surgical technique in individuals with chronic extensor mechanism deficiency. Twenty-eight individuals with chronic extensor mechanism deficiency (quadriceps tendon rupture $n = 9$, patellar tendon rupture $n = 19$) after TKA were analyzed. Surgical reconstruction was carried out with a monofilament polypropylene mesh (Marlex Mesh, Bard, Murray Hill, USA). The mean age at the time of surgery was 69 years. Individuals presented with a mean BMI of 33 kg/m^2. The mean follow-up period was 23 months. The 2-year survivorship free of mesh revision was 89%. Three individuals (11%) had to experience revision because of mechanical mesh failure and received another polypropylene mesh. No further revisions were carried out thereafter. Flexion was 87° on average. Most individuals (75%, 21/28) had a full active extension. The mean active extension lag after surgery was 4°. A significant improvement of extensor mechanism function was observed. Most individuals had full extension and demonstrated good clinical outcomes. A failure rate of over 50% has been published for alternative procedures. Therefore, the employment of the reported procedure represented a reasonable management alternative for chronic extensor mechanism disruptions of the patellar tendon as well as the quadriceps tendon after TKA. However, there may be a possibly higher risk for infection persistence in periprosthetic joint infection (PJI) cases because of the presence of a foreign material [21].

15.5 Medial Gastrocnemius Flap

A gastrocnemius flap might be needed for extensor mechanism reconstruction in cases where there is substantial bone loss of the proximal tibia, making Achilles tendon allograft and extensor mechanism allograft not plausible, or when additional soft tissue coverage is needed around the anterior aspect of the knee [22, 23]. The medial gastrocnemius muscle must be mobilized, leaving its proximal attachment. Then, it must be brought anteriorly to cover the anterior aspect of the knee and sutured onto the underlying tissue. Finally, the tendon end of the flap is repaired onto the quadriceps tendon [2, 23, 24]. Jaureguito et al. reported overall results with improvement in ROM and mobility and decrease in extensor lag [23]. In another study by Busfield et al., seven individuals had a mean extensor lag of 13.5° at an average of 21 months of follow-up. All individuals returned to independent mobility [24].

15.6 Comparative Studies

15.6.1 Synthetic Mesh Versus Allograft

In 2018, Shau et al. conducted a systematic review of the literature. They found that baseline demographics and patient complexity were similar between the two procedures (synthetic mesh and allograft). Reconstruction success rates (76% allograft versus 74% mesh), average time to diagnosis/treatment, KSS, knee ROM/extensor lag, and complication percentages were similar (no statistical difference). Synthetic mesh was employed more commonly with concomitant revision of components. This systematic review showed equivalent success of allograft and synthetic mesh with around 25% failure rate in both procedures. PJI remained a frequent and substantial adverse event and reason for failure in both techniques. Synthetic mesh demonstrated equivalent extensor mechanism reconstruction success as allograft but with much lower cost, near universal availability, lack of illness transmission, and potential for reducing graft stretch-out [25].

In a study with level 3 of evidence published in 2019 by Wood et al., they compared the results of extensor mechanism allograft with synthetic graft reconstruction. They analyzed 27 individuals. A substantially greater postoperative extensor lag was encountered in the allograft cohort. Graft failure following synthetic reconstruction was zero, with an overall revision surgery rate of 15%. Graft failure was 21%, and the revision surgery rate was 43% following allograft reconstruction. The allograft cost was substantially higher compared with the synthetic graft cost. Synthetic reconstruction for extensor mechanism disruption demonstrated benefit in postoperative extensor lag, graft failure, revision surgery, and cost when compared with allograft [26].

In a meta-analysis published in 2021 by 2021 Deren et al., they compared both allograft and synthetic reconstructive procedures for success, reoperation, and infection percentages and functional results. Thirty studies were included. The overall success rate of the reconstruction was 73.3%. The success percentage of allograft was not substantially different from synthetic material. There was no substantial difference in revision percentages between allograft and synthetic material. The overall relative risk of infection was 4.301. There was no substantial difference in relative risk of infection between allograft (3.886) and synthetic material (4.851). No statistically significant difference was encountered in mean postoperative KSS (73.109 versus 72.679) between allograft and mesh reconstruction cohorts. This study showed the difficulty in managing this severe injury, independent of technique, as well as the substantial risk for overall failure and infection [27].

In a study with level 3 of evidence published in 2023 by Gencarelli et al., they compared clinical results and survivorship between allograft and synthetic mesh for reconstruction of native extensor mechanism rupture following TKA. Individuals aged ≥45 years old with native extensor mechanism disruption treated with either allograft or synthetic mesh with minimum 2-year follow-up were included. Demographic information, injury mechanism, ROM, surgical time, revision surgeries, and postoperative Knee Injury and Osteoarthritis Outcome Scores (KOOS JR) were collected. The Kaplan-Meier survival curve method was utilized to determine the survivorship as treatment failure was defined as postoperative extensor mechanism lag >30° or revision surgery. Twenty individuals experienced extensor mechanism reconstruction utilizing allograft versus 35 with synthetic mesh. Both cohorts had similar demographics and an average follow-up time of 3.5 years. Individuals treated with allograft had substantially greater postoperative flexion than individuals treated with mesh (99.4 allograft versus 92.6 synthetic mesh). However, there was no difference in postoperative results between the two cohorts in average KOOS JR., extensor lag, graft failure, revision surgery rates, surgical time, or ambulatory status at the most recent follow-up. Survival curve comparison also yielded no difference at up to 5-year follow-up. The findings of this study suggested that reconstruction with allograft or synthetic mesh results in similar clinical results with good survivorship [28].

In 2023, Anderson et al. stated that extensor mechanism disruption after TKA is a devastating problem usually treated with allograft or synthetic reconstruction and that comprehending of reconstruction success percentages and patient recorded results was lacking. Individuals who had an extensor mechanism disruption following TKA experiencing mesh or whole-extensor allograft reconstruction, with minimum 2-year follow-up, were analyzed. Functional failure was defined as extensor lag >30°, amputation, or fusion, as well as revision extensor mechanism reconstruction. Survivorship was evaluated using Kaplan-Meier curves. Of 56 extensor mechanism reconstructions (49 individuals), 50% (28/56) were functionally successful at 3.2 years of mean follow-up. In situ survivorship of the reconstructions at 36 months was 75.0% (42 of 58). There were 50% (14 of 28) of functionally failed extensor mechanism reconstructions that retained their reconstruction at last follow-up. Mean extensor lag among successes and failures was 5.4° and 71°, respectively. Mean Knee Injury and Osteoarthritis Outcome Score, Joint Replacement, scores were 67.1 and 48.8 among successes and failures. There were 64% (16 of 25) of successes and 1 of 19 failures that obtained a Knee Injury and Osteoarthritis Outcome Score, Joint Replacement, score above the minimum patient-acceptable symptom state for TKA. Survivorship and success percentages were similar between reconstruction methods. All-cause mortality was 8.2% (4 of 49), each with extensor mechanism reconstruction failure before death. All-cause reoperation rate was 42.9% (24 of 56), with a 14.3% (8 of 56) rate of revision extensor mechanism reconstruction and 10.7% (6 of 56) rate of above-knee amputation or modular fusion. This study of mesh or allograft extensor mechanism reconstruction showed modest functional success at 3.2 years. Complication and reoperation percentages were high, regardless of extensor mechanism reconstruction procedure. Consequently, extensor mechanism disruption following TKA remains problematic [29].

15.6.2 Achilles Tendon Allograft with a Calcaneal Block Versus Autograft of the Quadriceps Tendon Reinforced by the Semitendinosus Tendon Versus a Full Extensor Mechanism Allograft Consisting of the Tibial Tubercle, Patellar Tendon, Patella, and Quadriceps Tendon

In a study with level 4 of evidence published in 2018 by Lamberti et al., they compared mid-run outcomes of three different reconstructive procedures for chronic patellar tendon disruption after TKA. Their hypothesis was that allografts provide better functional outcomes than autografts in restoring a correct joint function. Twenty-one reconstructions were carried out in twenty-one individuals (three cohorts of seven individuals) with chronic patellar tendon lesion after TKA. Cohort I experienced reconstruction with an Achilles tendon allograft with a calcaneal block, cohort II with an autograft of the quadriceps tendon reinforced by the semitendinosus tendon, and cohort III with a full extensor mechanism allograft consisting of the tibial tubercle, patellar tendon, patella, and quadriceps tendon. The mean extensor lag diminished from 50° to 3°. The KSS improved from 44.7 to 78.9 points. The comparison between the cohorts demonstrated statistically significant differences in the mean postoperative knee score between cohorts I (average score of 87.7 points) and II (average score of 70 points) but not between cohorts I and III (average score of 78.9 points) or between cohorts II and III. Differences in the postoperative extensor lag were not substantial between the three cohorts. According to this study, an Achilles tendon allograft should be considered the gold standard repair. The autograft technique is suitable when the host tissue is competent, particularly when dealing with younger individuals or postinfection. A full extensor mechanism allograft might represent a dependable solution when the defect involves the patellar bone or the quadriceps tendon [30].

15.7 Revision Extensor Mechanism Allograft (EMA) Reconstruction Following a Failed EMA

In 2023, Weintraub et al. stated that individuals who fail initial EMA reconstruction for extensor mechanism disruption after TKA are left with few alternatives. This study assessed results in individuals that experienced revision EMA reconstruction after a failed EMA. Ten individuals that experienced revision EMA for failed index EMA with minimum 1-year follow-up were analyzed. Individuals receiving fresh-frozen EMA (quadriceps tendon, patella, patellar tendon, and tibial tubercle) at index and revision EMA were included. The primary outcome was EMA failure defined as revision surgery, extensor lag >30°, or KSS <60 at last follow-up. Mean extensor lag improved from 55.6° pre-revision to 32.8° at mean follow-up of 43.8 months. Mean KSS improved from 41 pre-revision to 73.4 at last follow-up. All individuals needed assistive devices for ambulation at final follow-up: one (10%) needed a wheelchair, five (50%) needed a walker, and four (40%) needed a cane. Seven (70%) individual experienced EMA failure at a mean of 33.6 months following revision EMA: three (30%) were revised for PJI (one of which also had extensor lag >30°), three (30%) additional individuals had extensor lag >30°, and one (10%) individual had KSS <60 (this individual developed PJI and was treated nonoperatively with chronic antibiotic suppression). Revision EMA reconstruction fails at a high percentage in spite of leading to improvements in KSS. Further research is required to develop efficacious prevention and treatment approaches for failure after initial EMA reconstruction [31].

15.8 Conclusions

Reconstructive and augmentation alternatives for extensor mechanism failure after pTKA or rTKA comprise autograft, allograft, synthetic graft, and medial gastrocnemius flap. The semitendinosus autograft graft can only be utilized if the patella is not substantially retracted and there is good bone quality remaining in the patella. In a study, synthetic mesh demonstrated equivalent extensor mechanism reconstruction success as allograft but with much lower cost, near universal availability, lack of illness transmission, and potential for reducing graft stretch-out. Another study with a mean follow-up of 3.2 years compared mesh or allograft extensor mechanism reconstruction. All-cause reoperation rate was 42.9%, with a 14.3% rate of revision extensor mechanism reconstruction and 10.7% rate of above-knee amputation or modular fusion. Survivorship and success percentages were similar between reconstruction methods. Another study assessed results in individuals that experienced revision extensor mechanism allograft (EMA) reconstruction after a failed EMA. Revision EMA reconstruction failed at a high percentage. Extensor mechanism disruption following primary or revision TKA remains problematic.

References

1. Schoderbek RJ, Brown TE, Mulhall KJ, Mounasamy V, Iorio R, Krackow KA, et al. Extensor mechanism disruption after total knee arthroplasty. Clin Orthop Relat Res. 2006;446:176–85. https://doi.org/10.1097/01.blo.0000218726.06473.26.
2. Bates MD, Springer BD. Extensor mechanism disruption after total knee arthroplasty. J Am Acad Orthop Surg. 2015;23(2):95–106. https://doi.org/10.5435/JAAOS-D-13-00205.
3. Rosenberg AG. Management of extensor mechanism rupture after TKA. J Bone Joint Surg Br. 2012;94(11 Suppl A):116–9. https://doi.org/10.1302/0301-620X.94B11.30823.
4. Nam D, Abdel MP, Cross MB, LaMont LE, Reinhardt KR, McArthur BA, et al. The management of extensor mechanism complications in total knee arthroplasty: AAOS exhibit selection. J Bone Joint Surg Am. 2014;96(6):e47. https://doi.org/10.2106/JBJS.M.00949.
5. Ng J, Balcells-Nolla P, James PJ, Bloch BV. Extensor mechanism failure in total knee arthroplasty. EFORT Open Rev. 2021;6(3):181–8. https://doi.org/10.1302/2058-5241.6.200119.
6. Dobbs RE, Hanssen AD, Lewallen DG, Pagnano MW. Quadriceps tendon rupture after total knee arthroplasty: prevalence, complications, and outcomes. J Bone Joint Am. 2005;87(1):37–45. https://doi.org/10.2106/JBJS.D.01910.
7. Rand JA, Morrey BF, Bryan RS. Patellar tendon rupture after total knee arthroplasty. Clin Orthop Relat Res. 1989;244:233–8.

8. Cadambi A, Engh GA. Use of a semitendinosus tendon autogenous graft for rupture of the patellar ligament after total knee arthroplasty: a report of seven cases. J Bone Joint Surg Am. 1992;74(7):974–9.
9. Spoliti M, Giai Via A, Padulo J, Oliva F, Del Buono A, Maffulli N. Surgical repair of chronic patellar tendon rupture in total knee replacement with ipsilateral hamstring tendons. Knee Surg Sports Traumatol Arthrosc. 2016;24(10):3183–90. https://doi.org/10.1007/s00167-014-3448-9.
10. Takazawa Y, Ikeda H, Ishijima M, Kubota M, Saita Y, Kaneko H, et al. Reconstruction of a ruptured patellar tendon using ipsilateral semitendinosus and gracilis tendons with preserved distal insertions: two case reports. BMC Res Notes. 2013;6:361. https://doi.org/10.1186/1756-0500-6-361.
11. Masouros P, Papazotos N, Chatzipanagiotou G, Kourtzis D, Moustakalis I, Tzurbakis M. A staged procedure for the treatment of chronic patellar tendon ruptures after total knee arthroplasty. Eur J Orthop Surg Traumatol. 2023;33(4):1051–6. https://doi.org/10.1007/s00590-022-03251-w.
12. Emerson RH Jr, Head WC, Malinin TI. Reconstruction of patellar tendon rupture after total knee arthroplasty with an extensor mechanism allograft. Clin Orthop Relat Res. 1990;260:154–61.
13. Burnett RS, Berger RA, Della Valle CJ, Sporer SM, Jacobs JJ, Paprosky WG, Rosenberg AG. Extensor mechanism allograft reconstruction after total knee arthroplasty. J Bone Joint Surg Am. 2005;87 Suppl 1(Pt 2):175–94. https://doi.org/10.2106/JBJS.E.00442.
14. Malhotra R, Garg B, Logani V, Bhan S. Management of extensor mechanism deficit as a consequence of patellar tendon loss in total knee arthroplasty: a new surgical technique. J Arthroplast. 2008;23(8):1146–51. https://doi.org/10.1016/j.arth.2007.08.011.
15. Diaz-Ledezma C, Orozco FR, Delasotta LA, Lichstein PM, Post ZD, Ong AC. Extensor mechanism reconstruction with Achilles tendon allograft in TKA: results of an abbreviate rehabilitation protocol. J Arthroplast. 2014;29(6):1211–5. https://doi.org/10.1016/j.arth.2013.12.020.
16. Boettner F, Bou MJ. Achilles tendon allograft for augmentation of the Hanssen patellar bone grafting. Knee Surg Sports Traumatol Arthrosc. 2015;23(4):1035–8. https://doi.org/10.1007/s00167-014-2845-4.
17. Lim CT, Amanatullah DF, Huddleston JI 3rd, Harris AHS, Hwang KL, Maloney WJ, et al. Reconstruction of disrupted extensor mechanism after total knee arthroplasty. J Arthroplast. 2017;32(10):3134–40. https://doi.org/10.1016/j.arth.2017.05.005.
18. Helito CP, Mozella AP, Varone BB, Demange MK, Gobbi RG, Minamoto STN, et al. Extensor mechanism transplantation after knee prosthesis: 70-month follow-up. Acta Ortop Bras. 2022;30(spe1):e253424. https://doi.org/10.1590/1413-785220223001e253424.
19. Abdel MP, Pagnano MW, Perry KI, Hanssen AD. Extensor mechanism reconstruction with use of Marlex mesh. JBJS Essent Surg Tech. 2019;9(2):e21. https://doi.org/10.2106/JBJS.ST.18.00106.
20. Giuntoli M, Bonicoli E, Piolanti N, Ipponi E, Vigorito A, Marchetti S, et al. Which role for synthetic ligaments in the reconstruction of patellar tendon chronic rupture after TKA? Mid-term outcomes using LARS ligament. Acta Biomed. 2020;91(4):e2020113. https://doi.org/10.23750/abm.v91i4.9088.
21. Fuchs M, Gwinner C, Meissner N, Pfitzner T, Perka C, von Roth P. Therapy of chronic extensor mechanism deficiency after total knee arthroplasty using a monofilament polypropylene mesh. Front Surg. 2022;9:1000208. https://doi.org/10.3389/fsurg.2022.1000208.
22. Goldberg VM, Figgie HE III, Inglis AE, Figgie MP, Sobel M, Kelly M, et al. Patellar fracture type and prognosis in condylar total knee arthroplasty. Clin Orthop Relat Res. 1988;236:115–22.
23. Jaureguito JW, Dubois CM, Smith SR, Gottlieb LJ, Finn HA. Medial gastrocnemius transposition flap for the treatment of disruption of the extensor mechanism after total knee arthroplasty. J Bone Joint Surg Am. 1997;79(6):866–73. https://doi.org/10.2106/00004623-199706000-00010.
24. Busfield BT, Huffman GR, Nahai F, Hoffman W, Ries MD. Extended medial gastrocnemius rotational flap for treatment of chronic knee extensor mechanism deficiency in patients with

and without total knee arthroplasty. Clin Orthop Relat Res. 2004;428:190–7. https://doi.org/10.1097/01.blo.0000148593.44691.30.
25. Shau D, Patton R, Patel S, Ward L, Guild G 3rd. Synthetic mesh vs. allograft extensor mechanism reconstruction in total knee arthroplasty—a systematic review of the literature and meta-analysis. Knee. 2018;25(1):2–7. https://doi.org/10.1016/j.knee.2017.12.004.
26. Wood TJ, Leighton J, Backstein DJ, Marsh JD, Howard JL, McCalden RW, et al. Synthetic graft compared with allograft reconstruction for extensor mechanism disruption in total knee arthroplasty: a multicenter cohort study. J Am Acad Orthop Surg. 2019;27(12):451–7. https://doi.org/10.5435/JAAOS-D-18-00393.
27. Deren ME, Pannu TS, Villa JM, Firtha M, Riesgo AM, Higuera CA. Meta-analysis comparing allograft to synthetic reconstruction for extensor mechanism disruption after total knee arthroplasty. J Knee Surg. 2021;34(3):338–50. https://doi.org/10.1055/s-0039-1696656.
28. Gencarelli P Jr, Yawman JP, Tang A, Salandra J, North DD, Menken LG, et al. Extensor mechanism reconstruction after total knee arthroplasty with allograft versus synthetic mesh: a multicenter retrospective cohort. J Am Acad Orthop Surg. 2023;31(1):e23–34. https://doi.org/10.5435/JAAOS-D-22-00401.
29. Anderson JT, McLeod CB, Anderson LA, Pelt CE, Gililland JM, Peters CL, et al. Extensor mechanism disruption remains a challenging problem. J Arthroplast. 2023;38(6S):S337–44. https://doi.org/10.1016/j.arth.2023.03.067.
30. Lamberti A, Balato G, Summa PP, Rajgopal A, Vasdev A, Baldini A. Surgical options for chronic patellar tendon rupture in total knee arthroplasty. Knee Surg Sports Traumatol Arthrosc. 2018;26(5):1429–35. https://doi.org/10.1007/s00167-016-4370-0.
31. Weintraub MT, Bailey Terhune E, Serino J 3rd, Della Valle E, Della Valle CJ. High rate of failure after revision extensor mechanism allograft reconstruction. Knee. 2023;42:181–5. https://doi.org/10.1016/j.knee.2023.03.008.

Artificial Intelligence in Revision Total Knee Arthroplasty

E. Carlos Rodríguez-Merchán

16.1 Introduction

The contemporary employments of the virtual elements of artificial intelligence (AI), machine learning (ML), and deep learning (DL) in primary total knee arthroplasty (pTKA) are various. ML can foretell the length of stay (LOS) and costs prior to pTKA, the risk of transfusion after pTKA, postoperative dissatisfaction after pTKA, the size of pTKA components, and poorest results. The forecast of distinct results with ML models using specific information is already possible; nonetheless, the forecast of more complex outcomes is still imprecise. Remote patient monitoring systems present the capacity to more completely evaluate the individuals undergoing pTKA in terms of mobility and rehabilitation compliance. DL can precisely recognize the presence of pTKA, differentiate between specific arthroplasty designs, and recognize and classify knee osteoarthritis as precisely as an orthopedic surgeon. DL permits for the detection of prosthetic loosening from radiographs. Concerning the architectures associated with DL, artificial neural networks (ANN) and convolutional neural networks (CNN), ANN can foretell LOS, inpatient expenses, and discharge disposition before pTKA and CNN permit for differentiation between different implant types with near-perfect exactness [1, 2]. However, in a systematic review published in 2022 by Karlin et al., they stated that supervised ML algorithms should be critically evaluated and validated before clinical adoption [3]. The purpose of this chapter is to review recent developments on the role of artificial intelligence in revision total knee arthroplasty (rTKA).

E. C. Rodríguez-Merchán (✉)
Department of Orthopedic Surgery, La Paz University Hospital, Madrid, Spain

16.2 Machine-Learning (ML) Can Detect Prosthetic Loosening from Radiographs in First-Time rTKA with an Accuracy of About 86%

In 2020, Shah et al. evaluated the ability of an ML algorithm to diagnose prosthetic loosening from preoperative radiographs and investigated the inputs that might improve its performance. A cohort of 697 individuals experienced a first-time revision of a total hip (rTHA) or rTKA. Preoperative anteroposterior and lateral radiographs and historical and comorbidity data were collected from their electronic records. Each individual was defined as having loose or fixed components based on the operation notes. Shah et al. trained a series of CNN models to foretell a diagnosis of loosening at the time of surgery from the preoperative radiographs. They then added historical information about the individuals to the best performing model to produce a final model and tested it on an independent dataset. The CNN they constructed performed well when detecting loosening from radiographs alone. The first model built de novo with only the radiological image as input had an accuracy of 70%. The final model, which was constructed by fine-tuning a publicly accessible model named DenseNet, combining the AP and lateral radiographs, and incorporating data from the patient's history, had an accuracy, sensitivity, and specificity of 88.3%, 70.2%, and 95.6% on the independent test dataset. It performed better for individuals of rTHA with an accuracy of 90.1%, than for individuals of rTKA with an accuracy of 85.8%. This study demonstrated that ML can detect prosthetic loosening from radiographs. Its accuracy is improved when utilizing highly trained public algorithms and when adding clinical data to the algorithm [4].

16.3 Artificial Intelligence Algorithms for the Prediction of Nonhome Discharge Disposition for Individuals After rTKA

In a study with level 4 of evidence published in 2022 by Klemt et al., they developed and validated artificial intelligence algorithms to foretell discharge disposition following rTKA. A retrospective review of electronic patient records was carried out to recognize individuals who experienced rTKA. Discharge disposition was defined as either home discharge or nonhome discharge, which included rehabilitation and skilled nursing facilities. Four artificial intelligence algorithms were developed to foretell this result and were evaluated by discrimination, calibration, and decision curve analysis. A total of 2228 individuals experienced rTKA, of which 1405 individuals (63.1%) were discharged home, whereas 823 individuals (36.9%) were discharged to a nonhome facility. The strongest predictors for nonhome discharge after rTKA of this study are shown in Fig. 16.1. The best performing artificial intelligence algorithm was the neural network model which accomplished excellent performance across discrimination, calibration, and decision curve analysis. This study developed four artificial intelligence algorithms for the forecast of nonhome

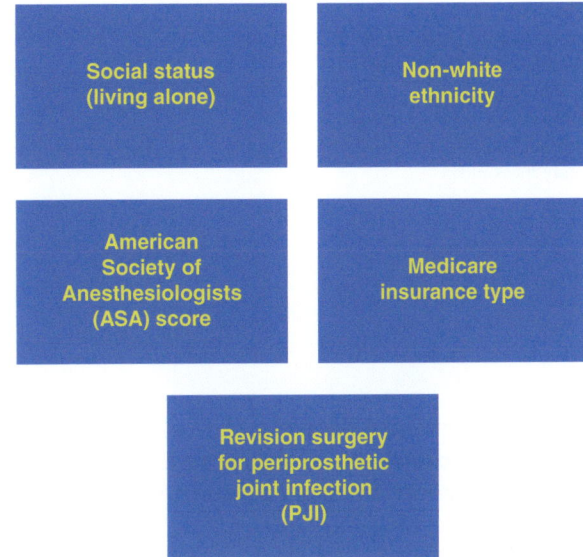

Fig. 16.1 Strongest predictors for nonhome discharge after revision total knee arthroplasty (rTKA) using artificial intelligence

discharge disposition for individuals after rTKA. The study showed excellent performance on discrimination, calibration, and decision curve analysis for all four candidate algorithms. Consequently, these models have the possibility to guide preoperative patient counselling and improve the value (clinical and functional results divided by costs) of rTKA individuals [5].

16.4 Artificial Intelligence Algorithms Predict Prolonged LOS Following rTKA

Klemt et al. developed and validated artificial intelligence algorithms for the forecast of prolonged LOS for individuals after rTKA in a study with level 4 of evidence published in 2022. A total of 2512 consecutive individuals who experienced rTKA were assessed. Those individuals with a LOS greater than 75th percentile for all LOSs were defined as individuals with prolonged LOS. Three artificial intelligence algorithms were developed to foretell prolonged LOS after rTKA, and these models were evaluated by discrimination, calibration, and decision curve analysis. The strongest predictors for prolonged LOS after rTKA of this study are shown in Fig. 16.2. The three artificial intelligence algorithms all accomplished excellent performance across discrimination and decision curve analysis. The study showed excellent performance on discrimination, calibration, and decision curve analysis for all three candidate algorithms. This highlighted the potential of these artificial intelligence algorithms to aid in the preoperative recognition of individuals with an increased risk of prolonged LOS after rTKA, which might assist in strategic discharge planning [6].

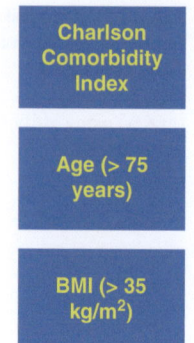

Fig. 16.2 Strongest predictors for prolonged length of stay (LOS) after revision total knee arthroplasty (rTKA) using artificial intelligence. BMI, body mass index

16.5 Machine-Learning Models Predict 30-Day Mortality, Cardiovascular Adverse Events, and Respiratory Adverse Events Following Aseptic rTKA

In a study with level 3 of evidence published in 2022 by Abraham et al., they studied whether ML can predict 30-day mortality and adverse events for individuals experiencing aseptic rTHA or rTKA and also what patient variables were the most relevant in forecasting adverse events. This was a temporally validated, retrospective study analyzing the 2014 to 2019 National Surgical Quality Improvement Program database, as this database captured a large group of aseptic rTKA individuals across a broad range of clinical settings and includes preoperative laboratory values. The training dataset was 2014 to 2018, and 2019 was the validation dataset. Given that predictive models learn expected prevalence of results, this split permits evaluation of model performance in contemporary individuals. Between 2014 and 2019, a total of 24,682 individuals experienced aseptic rTKA. This temporally validated model forecast 30-day mortality, cardiac adverse events, and respiratory adverse events following aseptic rTKA. This freely accessible risk calculator can be utilized preoperatively by surgeons to educate subjects on their individual postoperative risk of these specific adverse results [7].

16.6 Artificial Intelligence for the Prediction of PJI Following Aseptic rTKA

In 2023, Klemt et al. developed novel ML algorithms for the prediction of PJI after rTKA for individuals with aseptic indications for revision surgery. A single-institution database consisting of 1432 rTKA individuals with aseptic etiologies was identified. The patient group included 208 individuals (14.5%) who experienced re-revision surgery for PJI. Three ML algorithms (ANN, support vector machines, k-nearest neighbors) were developed to foretell this result, and these models were evaluated by discrimination, calibration, and decision curve analysis. Among the three ML models, the neural network model accomplished the best performance across discrimination, calibration, and decision curve analysis. The strongest predictors for PJI after rTKA for aseptic reasons were prior open procedure before revision surgery, drug abuse, obesity, and diabetes. This study used ML as a tool for the forecast of PJI following rTKA for aseptic failure with excellent performance. The validated ML models can help orthopedic surgeons in patient-specific risk stratifying to aid in preoperative counseling and clinical decision-making for individuals experiencing aseptic rTKA [8].

16.7 Machine-Learning Models Accurately Predict Recurrent Infection Following rTKA for PJI

In a study with level 4 of evidence published in 2022, Klemt et al. developed and validated ML models for the forecast of recurrent infection in individuals after rTKA for PJI. A total of 618 individuals experienced rTKA for PJI. The patient group included 165 individuals with confirmed recurrent PJI. Possible risk factors including patient demographics and surgical characteristics served as input to three ML models which were developed to forecast recurrent PJI. The ML models were evaluated by discrimination, calibration, and decision curve analysis. In this study, the factors most substantially associated with recurrent PJI in individuals following rTKA for PJI are shown in Fig. 16.3. The ML models all accomplished excellent performance across discrimination. This study developed three ML models for the

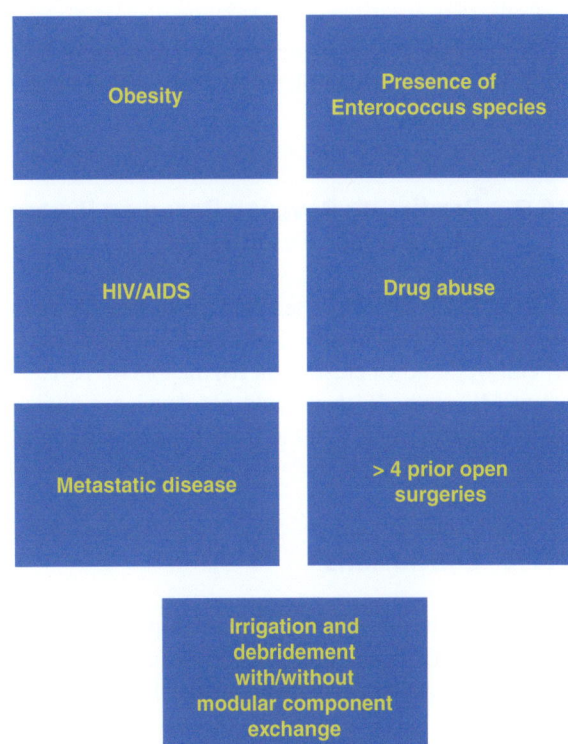

Fig. 16.3 Factors most substantially associated with recurrent periprosthetic joint infection (PJI) in individuals following revision total knee arthroplasty (rTKA) for PJI using artificial intelligence. HIV/AIDS, human immunodeficiency virus/acquired immunodeficiency syndrome

forecast of recurrent infections in individuals after rTKA for PJI. The strongest predictors were previous irrigation and debridement with or without modular component exchange and prior open surgeries [9].

16.8 Machine-Learning for the Prediction of Venous Thromboembolism and Major Bleeding Events Following rTKA

In 2023, Shohat et al. stated that venous thromboembolism (VTE) and major bleeding (MBE) are feared adverse events that are impacted by numerous host and surgical-related factors. Using ML on contemporary data, their objective was to develop and validate a practical, easy-to-use algorithm to foretell risk for VTE and MBE after total joint arthroplasty (TJA). This was a single institutional study of 35,963 primary and revision THA and TKA individuals. The group was divided to training (70%) and test (30%) sets. Four ML models were developed for each of the results evaluated (VTE and MBE). Models were generated for all VTE grouped together as well as for pulmonary emboli (PE) and deep vein thrombosis (DVT) individually to examine the need for distinct algorithms. For each result, the model that best performed utilizing repeated cross validation was chosen for algorithm development, and predicted versus observed incidences were assessed. Of the 35,963 individuals included, 308 (0.86%) developed VTE (170 PE's, 176 DVT's) and 293 (0.81%) developed MBE. Shohat et al. successfully developed and validated an easy-to-use algorithm that accurately foretells VTE and MBE after TJA. This tool can be utilized in every-day clinical decision-making and patient counseling [10].

16.9 Predicting Revision Based on Preoperative Information Alone Is Not Possible Yet

In 2020, El-Galaly et al. used the Danish Knee Arthroplasty Registry to build models to predict the likelihood of rTKA within 2 years of primary TKA. Although several well-known presurgical risk factors for revision were coupled with four different ML methods, they could not develop a clinically useful model capable of foretelling early rTKA in the Danish Knee Arthroplasty Registry based on preoperative information [11].

16.10 Conclusions

This chapter has reviewed recent developments on the role of artificial intelligence in rrTKA. ML can detect prosthetic loosening from radiographs in first-time rTKA with an accuracy of about 86%. Artificial intelligence algorithms predict prolonged

LOS following rTKA. ML models predict PJI following rTKA for aseptic failure, recurrent infection after rTKA for PJI, VTE and major bleeding events following rTKA, and 30-day mortality, cardiovascular adverse events, and respiratory adverse events after aseptic rTKA.

References

1. Rodriguez-Merchan EC. The current role of the virtual elements of artificial intelligence in total knee arthroplasty. EFORT Open Rev. 2022;7(7):491–7. https://doi.org/10.1530/EOR-21-0107.
2. Lau LCM, Chui ECS, Man GCW, Xin Y, Ho KKW, Mak KKK, et al. A novel image-based machine learning model with superior accuracy and predictability for knee arthroplasty loosening detection and clinical decision making. J Orthop Translat. 2022;36:177–83. https://doi.org/10.1016/j.jot.2022.07.004.
3. Karlin EA, Lin CC, Meftah M, Slover JD, Schwarzkopf R. The impact of machine learning on total joint arthroplasty patient outcomes: a systemic review. J Arthroplast. 2023;38(10):2085–95. https://doi.org/10.1016/j.arth.2022.10.039.
4. Shah RF, Bini SA, Martinez AM, Pedoia V, Vail TP. Incremental inputs improve the automated detection of implant loosening using machine-learning algorithms. Bone Joint J. 2020;102-B(6_Supple_A):101–6. https://doi.org/10.1302/0301-620X.102B6.BJJ-2019-1577.R1.
5. Klemt C, Uzosike AC, Harvey MJ, Laurencin S, Habibi Y, Kwon YM. Neural network models accurately predict discharge disposition after revision total knee arthroplasty? Knee Surg Sports Traumatol Arthrosc. 2022;30(8):2591–9. https://doi.org/10.1007/s00167-021-06778-3.
6. Klemt C, Tirumala V, Barghi A, Cohen-Levy WB, Robinson MG, Kwon YM. Artificial intelligence algorithms accurately predict prolonged length of stay following revision total knee arthroplasty. Knee Surg Sports Traumatol Arthrosc. 2022;30(8):2556–64. https://doi.org/10.1007/s00167-022-06894-8.
7. Abraham VM, Booth G, Geiger P, Balazs GC, Goldman A. Machine-learning models predict 30-day mortality, cardiovascular complications, and respiratory complications after aseptic revision total joint arthroplasty. Clin Orthop Relat Res. 2022;480(11):2137–45. https://doi.org/10.1097/CORR.0000000000002276.
8. Klemt C, Yeo I, Harvey M, Burns JC, Melnic C, Uzosike AC, et al. The use of artificial intelligence for the prediction of periprosthetic joint infection following aseptic revision total knee arthroplasty. J Knee Surg. 2023;37:158. https://doi.org/10.1055/s-0043-1761259. Online ahead of print.
9. Klemt C, Laurencin S, Uzosike AC, Burns JC, Costales TG, Yeo I, et al. Machine learning models accurately predict recurrent infection following revision total knee arthroplasty for periprosthetic joint infection. Knee Surg Sports Traumatol Arthrosc. 2022;30(8):2582–90. https://doi.org/10.1007/s00167-021-06794-3.
10. Shohat N, Ludwick L, Sherman MB, Fillingham Y, Parvizi J. Using machine learning to predict venous thromboembolism and major bleeding events following total joint arthroplasty. Sci Rep. 2023;13(1):2197. https://doi.org/10.1038/s41598-022-26032-1.
11. El-Galaly A, Grazal C, Kappel A, Nielsen PT, Jensen SL, Forsberg JA. Can machine-learning algorithms predict early revision TKA in the Danish Knee Arthroplasty Registry? Clin Orthop Relat Res. 2020;478(9):2088–101. https://doi.org/10.1097/CORR.0000000000001343.

Re-Revision Total Knee Arthroplasty

E. Carlos Rodríguez-Merchán

17.1 Introduction

According to Carr et al., approximately 20% of patients are unsatisfied with their postoperative outcomes following total knee arthroplasty (TKA). The main reasons for revision surgery are periprosthetic joint infection (PJI), aseptic loosing, instability, and malalignment. Much less commonly, secondary progression of patellar osteoarthritis, periprosthetic fractures, extensor mechanism insufficiency, polyethylene wear, and arthrofibrosis can require reintervention. Although detecting the cause of painful TKA can be difficult, it is a prerequisite for successful treatment [1].

Regarding the frequency of revision TKA, the most reported causes are aseptic loosening (29.8%), septic loosening (14.8%), pain (9.5%), wear (8.2%), and others [2]. It is important to note that all-cause revision rates following primary TKA double in patients with a body mass index (BMI) of 35 and over [3]. A retrospective study compared primary TKAs without previous surgery (group 1) with primary TKAs that had had previous arthroscopic debridement (group 2). After a minimum follow-up period of 2 years, previous knee arthroscopy showed a higher rate of failures [4].

It is important to note that in specialized arthroplasty hospitals, PJI was the most common reason for re-revision TKA [5]. Also, Halder et al. found evidence of a higher risk for re-revision surgery in hospitals with fewer than 25 revision TKAs per year [6].

The aim of this chapter was to assess the incidence, risk factors, and causes leading to re-revision TKA and the results (survivorship) of re-revision TKA.

E. C. Rodríguez-Merchán (✉)
Department of Orthopedic Surgery, La Paz University Hospital, Madrid, Spain

© The Author(s), under exclusive license to Springer Nature Switzerland AG 2024
E. C. Rodríguez-Merchán (ed.), *Advances in Revision Total Knee Arthroplasty*, https://doi.org/10.1007/978-3-031-60445-4_17

17.2 Incidence and Survival Rate of Re-Revision TKA

Infection is responsible for almost 50% of re-revision cases [7]. Several studies have demonstrated that the incidence of re-revision is depending on the number of previous surgeries and the preceding cause of revision [8–12].

For example, in aseptic revisions, the rate of re-revisions published by Bini et al. in 2016 was 10%, with a median time to reoperation of 3.6 years [8]. Regarding two-stage revision TKAs in infected TKA, Bongers et al. reported a 17% re-revision rate (11% due to infection and 6% for aseptic reasons) [9].

In cases of revision TKA for ligamentous instability treated with a mobile-bearing varus-valgus constrained (VVC) implant, a re-revision rate of 7% has been reported [10]. With regard to revision TKA with severe bone defects for which metaphyseal sleeves are required, the published re-revision rate has been 4% [11].

Re-revision rates reported by Meyer et al. in 2021 were between 4% and 10%, depending on the type of TKA revision performed (e.g., aseptic, septic, ligamentous instability, bone loss treated with metaphyseal sleeves) [12].

Early aseptic revision for pain within 90 days after primary TKA has been associated with higher odds of re-revision than early revisions performed for other causes (44% versus 29%) [13]. According to Kirschbaum et al., implant survivorship of re-revision TKA diminishes with an increasing number of revision surgeries [9]. In patients with severe arthrofibrosis revised with an RH prosthesis, implant survivorship free of any revision at 10 years was 54% in the RH cohort (versus 90% in the non-RH cohort) [14].

Chalmers et al. showed that, in 135 patients ≤50 years, implant survivorship free of all-cause re-revision was 66% at 10 years, with multiply revised TKAs having the poorest survival [15].

In 2021, Meyer et al. analyzed 235 aseptic revision TKAs: 14.8% underwent re-revision at mean follow-up of 8.3 years. Survivorship of re-revision TKA was 93% at 2 years and 83% at 8 years [8]. Patients with periprosthetic fractures around prior primary TKAs treated with distal femoral replacements with cemented femoral fixation had a 97% 5-year implant survivorship free from any re-revision [16].

In patients younger than 55 years who underwent aseptic revision TKA, implant survivorship free from any re-revision at 5 years was 80% [17]. In patients with idiopathic stiff TKA, isolated polyethylene exchange demonstrated re-revision percentages lower than component revision (16.7% versus 31%) [18].

17.3 Causes of Re-Revision TKA

Between 10% and 47.8% of the published TKA, re-revisions were due to PJI, between 14.3% and 21.9% due to aseptic loosening and between 13.7% and 25.7% due to periprosthetic fractures. Other percentages of interest regarding re-revision rates were 12% due to instability, 8% due to polyethylene wear, and 8% due to malpositioning of prosthetic components. Table 17.1 summarizes the main causes and rates of re-revision TKA in the literature [5, 12, 19–21].

Table 17.1 Causes for re-revision in the literature [5, 12, 19–21]

Authors [Reference]	Year	Number of cases	Follow-up period	Parameters	Conclusion
Postler et al. [5]	2018	These authors evaluated 312 individuals who experienced 402 revision TKA. In 289 individuals, this was the first revision surgery after primary TKA. Among the first revisions, the majority was late revisions (73.7%). One hundred and thirteen individuals (28.1%) had already had one or more revision surgeries before	NA	Revision causes were categorized utilizing all accessible data from patients' records including preoperative diagnostics, intraoperative findings, as well as the results of the periprosthetic tissue analysis	The most frequent reason for revision was PJI (36.1%) followed by aseptic loosening (21.9%) and periprosthetic fracture (13.7%)
Meyer et al. [12]	2021	235 aseptic revision TKAs were analyzed (14.8% experienced re-revision)	Mean follow-up: 8.3 years	Survivorship analysis	Survivorship of revision TKA was 93% at 2 years and 83% at 8 years. Average age at revision was 72.9 years. The most common reasons for failure following revision TKA were PJI (40%), periprosthetic fracture (25.7%), and aseptic loosening (14.3%). Of those whose revision TKA failed, the average survival was 3.33 years
Kirchsbaum et al. [19]	2022	Sixty-three patients (mean age 64 years) underwent 157 re-revision TKA surgeries (range 2–5)	Mean follow-up: 4.5 years	Survivorship analysis	The main reason for re-revision was PJI (48%), followed by instability (12%), polyethylene wear (11%), malpositioning (8%), and aseptic loosening (8%). Survivorship shortened with an increasing number of revision surgeries. While PJI was in 38% of all cases, the reason for the first revision, incidence increased constantly with the number of revisions (48% at second revision, 55% at third revision, 86% at fourth revision, and 100% at fifth revision. If PJI caused the first revision, patients showed an average of two more septic revisions at follow-up than patients with an aseptic first revision indication. In 36% of cases, the reason for follow-up surgery in case of PJI was again PJI

(continued)

Table 17.1 (continued)

Authors [Reference]	Year	Number of cases	Follow-up period	Parameters	Conclusion
Theil et al. [20]	2022	143 individuals who underwent revision TKA ($n = 119$) or complex primary TKA ($n = 24$) using a single-design condylar constrained knee system (Genesis CCK, Smith & Nephew) were analyzed	Mean follow-up: 11.8 years	Implant survivorship was analyzed using Kaplan-Meier survival estimates and multivariate Cox regression analysis to identify risk factors for failure	The implant survival was 86.4% after 5, 85.5% after 10, and 79.8% at 15 years. A reduced implant survivorship was found in males, smokers, and in obese patients. Patients who underwent primary TKA had a higher revision-free implant survivorship compared to revision TKA at 15 years (100% vs. 76%). The main cause for re-revision was infection in 10% of all revision TKA performed with the constrained condylar knee design included, while no case was revised for instability
van den Kieboom et al. [21]	2022	79 TKA patients underwent a revision for periprosthetic fracture, of which 15 TKA patients (18.9%) underwent re-revision surgery. The most common indication for knee re-revision was PJI in 11 TKA patients (47.8%).	Mean follow-up: 4.5 years	The complication rate of TKA revision was 25.3% and 39.1% for re-revision surgery. PJI was the most common indication for TKA re-revision (47.8%) and third revision surgery (13%). Factors contributing to an increased risk of TKA re-revision were revision with plate fixation and revision with combined ORIF	The most common indication for re-revision and third revision was PJI

PJI Periprosthetic joint infection, *ORIF* Open reduction and internal fixation

17.4 Risk Factors of Re-Revision TKA

Table 17.2 summarizes the main risk factors associated with re-revision TKA [6, 8, 13, 14, 16, 17, 21–26], considering patient-associated factors and procedure-associated factors.

Table 17.2 Main risk factors of re-revision total knee arthroplasty (TKA)

Patient-associated risk factors
Age was associated with a 20% lower risk for every 10-year increase [8]. Younger patients were at a higher risk of re-revision following aseptic revision TKA [23]. In hinge knee arthroplasty (HKA), male gender and younger age were independently associated with an augmented risk of re-revision [25]
Male patients were at a higher risk of re-revision following aseptic revision TKA [23]
Body mass index (BMI) was associated with a 20% lower risk for every 5-unit increase [8]
Patients with severe arthrofibrosis revised with a rotating hinge (RH) prosthesis were found to have a higher risk of re-revision than those in the non-RH cohort [14]
Smoking, right-sided TKA, and large femoral canal anteroposterior diameter were factors that augmented the risk of aseptic loosening after re-revision. Smokers had an 11.847-fold higher risk and right-sided TKA a 4.594-fold higher risk for aseptic loosening [22]
Patients who underwent early aseptic revision TKA within 90 days of surgery had a high risk of re-revision and infection at 2 years. Two-year survivorship free from additional revision surgery was inferior in the early aseptic revision group compared with the control (78% versus 98%). Among early revisions, 10% of the patients experienced re-revision for PJI, with an antibiotic spacer within 2 years [13]
Patients who had prior knee arthroscopy demonstrated a substantially higher probability of needing re-revision compared with patients who underwent revision TKA without prior knee arthroscopy. There was also a significantly augmented probability of re-revision in patients who had prior knee arthroscopy within 6 months [24]
Procedure-associated risk factors
In aseptic revisions, antibiotic-loaded cement was associated with a 50% lower risk of all-cause re-revision surgery [8]
Surgeon's greater cumulative experience (≥ 20 cases vs. <20 cases) was associated with a three times lower risk of re-revision [8]
Low hospital volume augmented the re-revision percentage after aseptic revision TKA. They found evidence of a higher risk for re-revision surgery in hospitals with fewer than 25 revision TKAs per year. Hospital volume had a substantial effect on the 1-year re-revision percentage [6]
Tibial tantalum cone was a factor that diminished the risk of aseptic loosening after re-revision. The presence of a tibial tantalum cone was associated with an 8.403-fold lower risk [22]
Distal femoral replacements (DFRs) for periprosthetic femur fractures around revision TKAs or conversions of failed open reduction and internal fixations (ORIFs) had a 5× increased risk of re-revision [16]
In patients younger than 55 years who underwent aseptic revision TKA, prior revision, an isolated polyethylene exchange, and an RH prosthesis were significant risk factors for shorter revision-free implant survival [17]
The likelihood of survival of the implanted TKA was substantially diminished with each subsequent revision [13]
In patients with periprosthetic fractures treated with revision TKA, factors significantly contributing to an augmented risk of TKA re-revision were revision with plate fixation and revision with combined ORIF [21]

Table 17.2 (continued)

Patient-associated risk factors
In HKA revision for PJI or implant fracture, a fixed hinge, or surgery carried out by a non-consultant grade were independently associated with an augmented risk of re-revision [25]
PJI, greater number of prior surgical procedures, and higher Elixhauser score were independently related to further surgery [26]

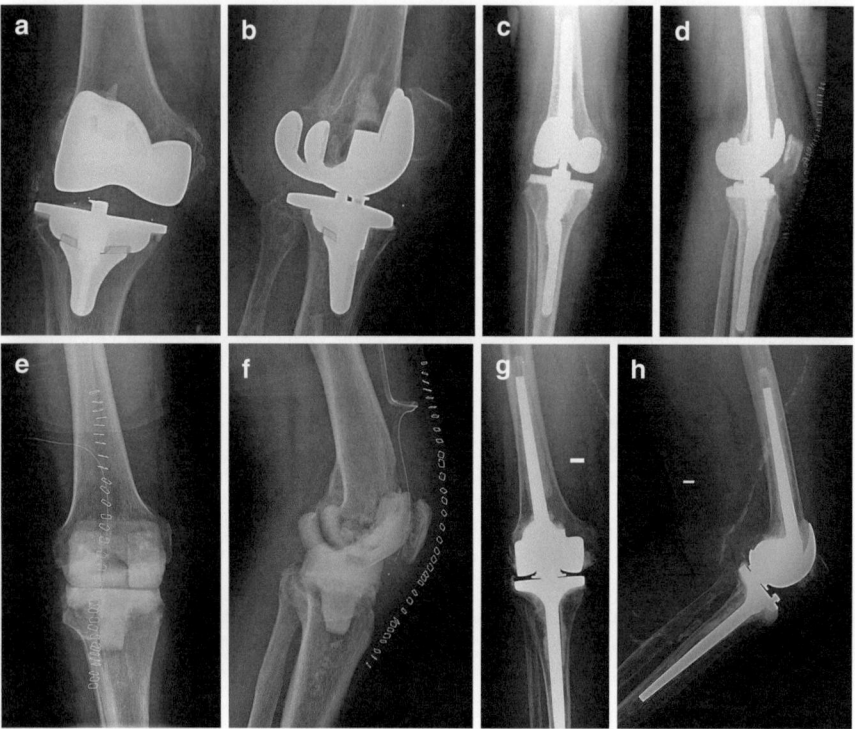

Fig. 17.1 (**a–h**) Two-stage re-revision total knee arthroplasty (TKA) with a rotating hinge (RH) implant due to periprosthetic joint infection (PJI) of a constrained condylar knee (CCK) prosthesis that was implanted after aseptic loosening of the initial implant: (**a**) anteroposterior (AP) view of the initial prosthesis; (**b**) lateral radiograph of the initial prosthesis; (**c**) AP view after revision TKA with the CCK design; (**d**) lateral radiograph after revision TKA with the CCK design; (**e**) AP view after removal of the infected CCK prosthesis and implantation of an articulated spacer; (**f**) lateral radiograph after removal of the infected CCK prosthesis and implantation of an articulated spacer; (**g**) AP view after second stage of re-revision with an RH design; (**h**) lateral radiograph after second stage of re-revision with an RH design

17.5 Results of Re-Revision TKA

Figure 17.1 shows a two-stage re-revision TKA with a rotating hinge (RH) implant due to PJI of a constrained condylar knee (CCK) prosthesis that was implanted after aseptic loosening of the initial implant, with a satisfactory result.

17.5.1 Re-Revision TKA Employing Fully Cemented Stems Carried Out on Femurs with Diaphyseal Deformity

In the study of Song et al., the 5- and 10-year survival rates were 100% and 93.2%, respectively. It seemed that fully cemented stems are viable in yielding long-run satisfactory survival after re-revision TKA in individuals with femoral diaphyseal deformity. However, it should be employed carefully for those with prior infections [27].

17.6 Re-Revision Due to PJI

17.6.1 Diagnosing PJI in Individuals Experiencing Re-Revision TKA

Xu et al. found that plasma levels of D-dimer and fibrin degradation product (FDP) might be inadequate for diagnosing PJI in individuals experiencing re-revision TKA, but the combination of serum CRP and interleukin-6 might be efficacious [28].

17.6.2 Timing of DAIR for Early Postsurgical Knee PJI Does Not Influence 1-Year Re-Revision Percentages

Van der Ende et al. found no substantial difference in 1-year re-revision percentage following a debridement, antibiotics, and implant retention (DAIR) procedure by timing of the DAIR procedure [29].

17.6.3 The Risk of Re-Revision Is Similar Between Single- and Two-Stage Revision for Infected Primary TKA

According to Lenguerrand et al., the risk of re-revision was alike between single- and two-stage revision for infected primary TKA. Single-stage patients needed fewer revisions. The single-stage revision was a safe and efficacious approach to manage infected TKAs [30].

17.6.4 Repeat Two-Stage Exchange Arthroplasty for PJI Is Dependent on Host Grade

Fehring et al. found that uncompromised hosts (MSIS type A) with an acceptable wound (MSIS type 1 or 2) had a 70% rate of success following a repeat two-stage exchange TKA, but type B2 hosts had a 50% success rate. The repeat two-stage exchange procedure failed in type-C3 hosts; consequently, alternative salvage procedures should be deemed for such individuals [31].

17.6.5 The Efficacy of Repeat Two-Stage Revision for the Treatment of Recalcitrant TKA Infection

According to Vaniee et al., another two-stage revision TKA was an efficacious method of treatment. However, Vadiee et al. found a higher prevalence of failure in those individuals with poor general health based on the MSIS score, inappropriate soft tissue envelope, and resistant bacteria. The success of second, two-stage procedure was best in individuals with optimized general health, soft tissue coverage, and antibiotic-sensitive bacteria. Individuals who cannot be optimized are most likely to need amputation or knee fusion than another futile two-stage procedure [32].

17.6.6 High Revision Percentages After Repeat Septic Revision Following Failed One-Stage Exchange for PJI in TKA

In 2022, Neufeld et al. stated that repeat septic revision after a failed one-stage exchange TKA for PJI was related to an elevated percentage of subsequent infection-related failure and all-cause revision. However, the host and limb status according to the MSIS system were not related to a subsequent infection-related failure [33].

17.6.7 Repeat Two-Stage Revision for PJI in TKA Leads to Very High Failure Percentages

Christener et al. showed that individuals experiencing a repeat two-stage TKA had very poor results. However, their study did not reveal any factors that foretold failure. Individuals must be counselled regarding poor results with repeat two-stage TKA, and other treatment alternatives such as early amputation or lifelong suppression should be deemed [34].

17.6.8 Repeat Revision TKA for Failed Management of PJI Has Long-Run Success but Frequently Needs Multiple Operations

In the study of Rajgor et al., successful eradication of infection was accomplished in 50% of individuals following re-revision surgery, compared with 91% following two-stage exchange of primary TKA for PJI [35].

17.7 Conclusions

After aseptic revision TKA, PJI and periprosthetic fracture are the main causes of re-revision surgery. In aseptic revisions, the use of antibiotic-loaded cement is associated with lower risk of re-revision. Patients younger than 50 years experiencing contemporary aseptic revision TKA have a one in three risk of re-revision. Acute early aseptic revision (within 90 days of surgery) TKA carries a high risk of re-revision at 2 years and a high risk of subsequent PJI. PJI is the most common reason for re-revision, third revision TKA, and multiple revisions. Patients specifically revised for instability or who had prior TKA revisions had the highest risk of re-revision at 10 years. The likelihood of implanted TKA survival is substantially diminished with each subsequent revision.

References

1. Carr AJ, Robertsson O, Graves S, Price AJ, Arden NK, Judge A, et al. Knee replacement. Lancet. 2012;379(9823):1331–40. https://doi.org/10.1016/S0140-6736(11)60752-6.
2. Sadoghi P, Liebensteiner M, Agreiter M, Leithner A, Böhler N, Labek G. Revision surgery after total joint arthroplasty: a complication-based analysis using worldwide arthroplasty registers. J Arthroplast. 2013;28(8):1329–32. https://doi.org/10.1016/j.arth.2013.01.012.
3. Zingg M, Miozzari HH, Fritschy D, Hoffmeyer P, Lübbeke A. Influence of body mass index on revision rates after primary total knee arthroplasty. Int Orthop. 2016;40(4):723–9. https://doi.org/10.1007/s00264-015-3031-0.
4. Piedade SR, Pinaroli A, Servien E, Neyret P. Is previous knee arthroscopy related to worse results in primary total knee arthroplasty? Knee Surg Sports Traumatol Arthrosc. 2009;17(4):328–33. https://doi.org/10.1007/s00167-008-0669-9.
5. Postler A, Lützner C, Beyer F, Tille E, Lützner J. Analysis of total knee arthroplasty revision causes. BMC Musculoskelet Disord. 2018;19(1):55. https://doi.org/10.1186/s12891-018-1977-y.
6. Halder AM, Gehrke T, Günster C, Heller KD, Leicht H, Malzahn J, et al. Low hospital volume increases re-revision rate following aseptic revision total knee arthroplasty: an analysis of 23,644 cases. J Arthroplast. 2020;35(4):1054–9. https://doi.org/10.1016/j.arth.2019.11.045.
7. Martinez R, Chen AF. Outcomes in revision in knee arthroplasty: preventing reoperation for infection keynote lecture—BASK annual congress 2023. Knee. 2023;43:A5–A10. https://doi.org/10.1016/j.knee.2023.07.010.
8. Bini SA, Chan PH, Inacio MC, Paxton EW, Khatod M. Antibiotic cement was associated with half the risk of re-revision in 1,154 aseptic revision total knee arthroplasties. Acta Orthop. 2016;87(1):55–9. https://doi.org/10.3109/17453674.2015.1103568.
9. Bongers J, Jacobs AME, Smulders K, van Hellemondt GG, Goosen JHM. Reinfection and re-revision rates of 113 two-stage revisions in infected TKA. J Bone Jt Infect. 2020;5(3):137–44. https://doi.org/10.7150/jbji.43705.
10. Reina N, Salib CG, Pagnano MW, Trousdale RT, Abdel MP, Berry DJ. Varus-valgus constrained implants with a mobile-bearing articulation: results of 367 revision total knee arthroplasties. J Arthroplast. 2020;35(4):1060–3. https://doi.org/10.1016/j.arth.2019.11.023.
11. Bonanzinga T, Akkawi I, Zahar A, Gehrke T, Haasper C, Marcacci M. Are metaphyseal sleeves a viable option to treat bone defect during revision total knee arthroplasty? A systematic review. Joints. 2019;7(1):19–24. https://doi.org/10.1055/s-0039-1697611.
12. Meyer JA, Zhu M, Cavadino A, Coleman B, Munro JT, Young SW. Infection and periprosthetic fracture are the leading causes of failure after aseptic revision total knee arthroplasty. Arch Orthop Trauma Surg. 2021;141(8):1373–83. https://doi.org/10.1007/s00402-020-03698-8.
13. Shen TS, Gu A, Bovonratwet P, Ondeck NT, Sculco PK, Su EP. Patients who undergo early aseptic revision TKA within 90 days of surgery have a high risk of re-revision and infection at 2 years: a large-database study. Clin Orthop Relat Res. 2022;480(3):495–503. https://doi.org/10.1097/CORR.0000000000001985.

14. Bingham JS, Bukowski BR, Wyles CC, Pareek A, Berry DJ, Abdel MP. Rotating-hinge revision total knee arthroplasty for treatment of severe arthrofibrosis. J Arthroplast. 2019;34(7S):S271–6. https://doi.org/10.1016/j.arth.2019.01.072.
15. Chalmers BP, Pallante GD, Sierra RJ, Lewallen DG, Pagnano MW, Trousdale RT. Contemporary revision total knee arthroplasty in patients younger than 50 years: 1 in 3 risk of re-revision by 10 years. J Arthroplast. 2019;34(7S):S266–70. https://doi.org/10.1016/j.arth.2019.02.001.
16. Chalmers BP, Syku M, Gausden EB, Blevins JL, Mayman DJ, Sculco PK. Contemporary distal femoral replacements for supracondylar femoral fractures around primary and revision total knee arthroplasties. J Arthroplast. 2021;36(7S):S351–7. https://doi.org/10.1016/j.arth.2020.12.037.
17. Chalmers BP, Syku M, Joseph AD, Mayman DJ, Haas SB, Blevins JL. High rate of re-revision in patients less than 55 years of age undergoing aseptic revision total knee arthroplasty. J Arthroplast. 2021;36(7):2348–52. https://doi.org/10.1016/j.arth.2020.12.008.
18. Xiong L, Klemt C, Yin J, Tirumala V, Kwon YM. Outcome of revision surgery for the idiopathic stiff total knee arthroplasty. J Arthroplast. 2021;36(3):1067–73. https://doi.org/10.1016/j.arth.2020.09.005.
19. Kirschbaum S, Erhart S, Perka C, Hube R, Thiele K. Failure analysis in multiple TKA revisions-periprosthetic infections remain surgeons' nemesis J Clin Med 2022;11(2):376. doi: https://doi.org/10.3390/jcm11020376.
20. Theil C, Schwarze J, Gosheger G, Poggenpohl L, Ackmann T, Moellenbeck B, et al. Good to excellent long-term survival of a single-design condylar constrained knee arthroplasty for primary and revision surgery. Knee Surg Sports Traumatol Arthrosc. 2022;30(9):3184–90. https://doi.org/10.1007/s00167-021-06636-2.
21. van den Kieboom J, Tirumala V, Xiong L, Klemt C, Kwon YM. Periprosthetic joint infection is the main reason for failure in patients following periprosthetic fracture treated with revision arthroplasty. Arch Orthop Trauma Surg. 2022;142(12):3565–74. https://doi.org/10.1007/s00402-021-03948-3.
22. Levent A, Suero EM, Gehrke T, Bakhtiari IG, Citak M. Risk factors for aseptic loosening in complex revision total knee arthroplasty using rotating hinge implants. Int Orthop. 2021;45(1):125–32. https://doi.org/10.1007/s00264-020-04878-2.
23. Klasan A, Magill P, Frampton C, Zhu M, Young SW. Factors predicting repeat revision and outcome after aseptic revision total knee arthroplasty: results from the New Zealand Joint Registry Knee Surg Sports Traumatol Arthrosc 2021;29(2):579–585. doi: https://doi.org/10.1007/s00167-020-05985-8.
24. Oganesyan R, Klemt C, Esposito J, Tirumala V, Xiong L, Kwon YM. Knee arthroscopy prior to revision TKA is associated with increased re-revision for stiffness. J Knee Surg. 2022;35(11):1223–8. https://doi.org/10.1055/s-0040-1722662.
25. Clement ND, Avery P, Mason J, Baker PN, Deehan DJ. First-time revision knee arthroplasty using a hinged prosthesis: temporal trends, indications, and risk factors associated with re-revision using data from the National Joint Registry for 3,855 patients. Bone Joint J. 2023;105-B(1):47–55. https://doi.org/10.1302/0301-620X.105B1.BJJ-2022-0522.R1.
26. von Fritsch L, Sabah SA, Xu J, Price AJ, Merle C, Alvand A. Re-revision knee arthroplasty in a tertiary center: infection and multiple previous surgeries were associated with poor early clinical and functional outcomes. J Arthroplast. 2023;38(7):1313–9. https://doi.org/10.1016/j.arth.2023.01.030.
27. Song SJ, Le HW, Bae DK, Park CH. Long-term survival of fully cemented stem in re-revision total knee arthroplasty performed on femur with diaphyseal deformation due to implant loosening. Int Orthop. 2022;46(7):1521–7. https://doi.org/10.1007/s00264-022-05412-2.
28. Xu H, Xie J, Wang D, Huang Q, Huang Z, Zhou Z. Plasma levels of D-dimer and fibrin degradation product are unreliable for diagnosing periprosthetic joint infection in patients undergoing re-revision arthroplasty. J Orthop Surg Res. 2021;16(1):628. https://doi.org/10.1186/s13018-021-02764-0.
29. van der Ende B, van Oldenrijk J, Reijman M, Croughs PD, van Steenbergen LN, Verhaar JAN, et al. Timing of debridement, antibiotics, and implant retention (DAIR) for early post-surgical

hip and knee prosthetic joint infection (PJI) does not affect 1-year re-revision rates: data from the Dutch Arthroplasty Register. J Bone Jt Infect. 2021;6(8):329–36. https://doi.org/10.5194/jbji-6-329-2021.
30. Lenguerrand E, Whitehouse MR, Kunutsor SK, Beswick AD, Baker RP, Rolfson O, et al. National Joint Registry for England, Wales, Northern Ireland and the Isle of Man. Mortality and re-revision following single-stage and two-stage revision surgery for the management of infected primary knee arthroplasty in England and Wales: evidence from the National Joint Registry. Bone Joint Res. 2022;11(10):690–9. https://doi.org/10.1302/2046-3758.1110.BJR-2021-0555.R1.
31. Fehring KA, Abdel MP, Ollivier M, Mabry TM, Hanssen AD. Repeat two-stage exchange arthroplasty for periprosthetic knee infection is dependent on host grade. J Bone Joint Surg Am. 2017;99(1):19–24. https://doi.org/10.2106/JBJS.16.00075.
32. Vadiee I, Backstein DJ. The effectiveness of repeat two-stage revision for the treatment of recalcitrant total knee arthroplasty infection. J Arthroplast. 2019;34(2):369–74. https://doi.org/10.1016/j.arth.2018.10.021.
33. Neufeld ME, Liechti EF, Soto F, Linke P, Busch S-M, Gehrke T, et al. High revision rates following repeat septic revision after failed one-stage exchange for periprosthetic joint infection in total knee arthroplasty. Bone Joint J. 2022;104-B(3):386–93. https://doi.org/10.1302/0301-620X.104B3.BJJ-2021-0481.R2.
34. Christiner T, Yates P, Prosser G. Repeat two-stage revision for knee prosthetic joint infection results in very high failure rates. ANZ J Surg. 2022;92(3):487–92. https://doi.org/10.1111/ans.17446.
35. Rajgor H, Dong H, Nandra R, Parry M, Stevenson J, Jeys L. Repeat revision TKR for failed management of peri-prosthetic infection has long-term success but often require multiple operations: a case control study. Arch Orthop Trauma Surg. 2023;143(2):987–94. https://doi.org/10.1007/s00402-022-04594-z.

If you have any concerns about our products,
you can contact us on
ProductSafety@springernature.com

In case Publisher is established outside the EU,
the EU authorized representative is:
Springer Nature Customer Service Center GmbH
Europaplatz 3, 69115 Heidelberg, Germany

Printed by Libri Plureos GmbH
in Hamburg, Germany